This edition of this book has b⟨…⟩restricted educational grant from Pfizer Limited.

D0414071

Other books by the same authors
(all from Oxford University Press)

# Bandolier's Evidence-based resource for Erectile dysfunction

Andrew Moore
Sheena Derry
Henry McQuay

Pain Research
Churchill Hospital
Oxford

A *Bandolier* book
Oxford

## Bandolier books

Bandolier books are published by Bandolier Ltd

Bandolier's Internet site is at www.ebandolier.com

Published in the United Kingdom
by Bandolier Ltd

British Library cataloguing in Publication Data
Data available

ISBN-10  0-9552226-0-5
ISBN-13  978-0-955226-0-3

Typeset in Minion
Cover design by Gwilym Johnson
Printed in Oxford, UK

# CONTENTS

# SECTION 1

# INTRODUCTION

This book was written as a simple guide for people who wish to make sense of evidence relating to erectile dysfunction, and the many different therapies that are now available. The book is not a comprehensive manual for diagnosis and treatment of erectile dysfunction, but a resource. The evidence will obviously change as more trials and new interventions appear, but for PDE-5 inhibitors, where there is already considerable evidence, much change is unlikely.

The reader will see reference to Bandolier at various parts of the book. That's because the authors write Bandolier, an independent journal about evidence-based healthcare, published since February 1994 in print and on the web (www.ebandolier.com), and we use examples from Bandolier in this book.

Bandolier seeks information about evidence of effectiveness (or lack of it) in systematic reviews, meta-analyses, randomised trials, and from high quality observational studies. This book is a summary of the tools that Bandolier uses to assess evidence, to be able to distinguish good evidence from bad. We have an adage that we advocate tools not rules, because we hope to stimulate thought, debate and innovation rather than to stifle.

These days everything is seemingly badged as "evidence-based", irrespective of the amount or quality of evidence that is available. Too often someone will claim an evidence base when the evidence they have is a study of two men and a dog, in which the dog got better and the men weren't ill anyway. Being evidence-based is actually rather more than that. It should mean that there is a minimum amount of good quality evidence, from valid studies, and free from bias.

Finding evidence to fit the bill is rather difficult. Consider the quotation by Richard Smith of some words of David Eddy, an important original thinker about evidence, in 1991:

*"There are perhaps 30000 biomedical journals in the world, and they have grown steadily by 7% a year since the seventeenth century. Yet about 15% of medical interventions are supported by solid scientific evidence......only 1% of the articles in medical journals are scientifically sound"* [1].

Bandolier's experience of reading lots of papers and systematic reviews over the past few decades is that this is not far from the truth. For instance, some of our own work has identified that in some cases 1 in 10 trial reports contain serious errors (actually 2 in 13 [2]), and others have also found similar problems.

### FAILURE OF PEER REVIEW

Most of us think that the peer review process in journals should protect us, from mistakes, from inaccurate or inadequate conclusions, or even from fraud. It does not. Peer reviewers are usually busy people, who try to help editors, their professional colleagues, and authors of papers by giving freely of their time to judge manuscripts, and to improve them. Many of us who write papers are grateful to reviewers who have helped improve our papers. But just as often unthinking, ignorant or insulting remarks by reviewers drive us to fury.

All too often accepting or rejecting submitted papers seems to be little less than the random play of chance. A study in neuroscience confirms just that [3]. Two journals that routinely sent manuscripts to two reviewers allowed access to the assessments of these manuscripts. One journal provided information on all manuscripts over a six-month period (179), and the other provided information on 116 consecutive manuscripts. Both journals used a structured assessment, and assessors were asked to make the judgements: should the manuscript be accepted, revised, or rejected, and was the priority for publication low, medium or high?

Agreement between reviewers was assessed using the kappa statistic. A value of 0 represents chance agreement, and a value of 1 perfect agreement. Scores of 0 to 0.2 are considered very poor, those between 0.2 and 0.4 poor, between 0.4 and 0.6 moderate, between 0.6 and 0.8 good and between 0.8 and 1 excellent. Agreement was less than good, and was not convincingly better than chance for either journal for acceptance, revision or rejection, or high, medium or low priority.

## PROBLEM OF BELIEF

It is all too easy to say that we "know" a treatment works because we have seen the benefits for patients who have had the treatment. All too often, these beliefs can be exploded when good clinical studies that meet minimal rules of evidence are performed. An example is the use of hyperbaric oxygen for multiple sclerosis. A systematic review [4] showed that:

- Four case series all showed benefit
- One non-randomised comparative study showed benefit
- 12 randomised trials, of which not one showed anything other than trivial benefit

The benefit seen in studies whose design leaves them open to bias was not seen in studies of more rigorous design. This happens frequently.

## BUSY PEOPLE

We are all busy people. In primary care in Europe, physicians have, on average, only a few minutes to spend with each patient [5]. Nor is it so very different in hospitals, or with different professions, so there is precious little time to spare on evidence.

We all have different backgrounds and experience. Some of us have spent many years doing research, exploring the bounds of our personal and corporate ignorance. Those who spend their lives doing research find it hard to take new findings on board, especially if there are methodological or statistical issues. Bandolier is reminded of a (clever) mathematician friend who gave a talk, full of symbols and equations. At best we saw through a glass darkly, and praised his ability to handle mathematics with such facility. His response was heartening, that when faced with new concepts and equations, it took him three years or so to become comfortable with them! What chance do we ordinary mortals have?

Most of us do not do research, or have never done research. Not having done research at any deep level or for any prolonged time is the common experience, probably of about 99% of healthcare professionals. Yet we are exhorted to include best research findings into our practice. Most of us just do not have the time to wade through long and complicated scientific papers, even if we had the skills to do so, so we just read the abstract to get the gist of what a paper says, and trust peer-review to eliminate the rubbish.

## Being cautious

There are many traps and pitfalls to negotiate when assessing evidence, and it is all too easy to be misled by an apparently beautiful study that later turns out to be wrong, or by a meta-analysis with impeccable credentials that seems to be trying to pull the wool over our eyes. Although these are themes often found in the pages of Bandolier, a little reinforcement rarely comes amiss.

### Law of initial results

So often early promising results are followed by others that are less impressive. It is almost as if there is a law that states that first results are always spectacular, and subsequent ones are mediocre: the law of initial results. It now seems [6], that there may be some truth in this.

Three major general medical journals (New England Journal of Medicine, JAMA, and Lancet) were searched for studies with more than 1000 citations published between 1990 and 2003. This is an extraordinarily high number of citations when you think that most papers are cited once if at all, and that a citation of more than a few hundred times is as rare as hens' teeth.

Of the 115 articles published, 49 were eligible for the study because they were reports of original clinical research (like tamoxifen for breast cancer prevention, or stent versus balloon angioplasty). Studies had sample sizes as low as 9 (nine) and as high as 87,000. There were two case series and four cohort studies, and 43 randomised trials. The randomised trials were very varied in size, though, from 146 to 29,133 subjects (median 1817 subjects; Figure 1.1). Fourteen of the 43 randomised trials (33%) had fewer than 1000 patients and 25 (58%) had fewer than 2,500 patients.

Of the 49 studies, seven were contra-dicted by later research. These seven contradicted studies included one case series with nine patients, three cohort studies with 40,000 to 80,000 patients, and three randomised trials, with 200, 875 and 2002 patients respectively. So only three of 43 randomised trials were contradicted (7%), compared with half the case series and three out of four cohort studies.

Figure 1.1: Size of highly-cited RCTs

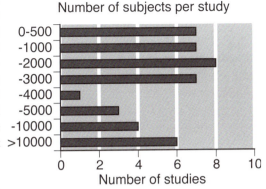

A further seven studies found effects stronger than subsequent research. One of these was a cohort study with 800 patients. The other six were randomised trials, four with fewer than 1000 patients and two with about 1500 patients.

Most of the observational studies had been contradicted, or subsequent research had shown substantially smaller effects, but most randomised studies had results that had not been challenged. Of the nine randomised trials that were challenged, six had fewer than 1000 patients, and all had fewer than 2003 patients. Of 23 randomised trials with 2002 patients or fewer, 9 were contradicted or challenged. None of the 20 randomised studies with more than 2003 patients were challenged.

## MOST PUBLISHED RESEARCH FALSE?

As we mentioned earlier, it has been suggested that only 1% of articles in scientific jour-nals are scientifically sound [1]. Bandolier has often examined articles showing how we consumers of scientific literature can be misled, and how we often are. Another paper from Greece [7] is replete with Greek mathematical symbols and philosophy. It makes a number of important points:

1. The smaller the studies conducted in a scientific field, the less likely the research find-ings are to be true.
2. The smaller the effect sizes in a scientific field, the less likely the research findings are to be true.
3. The greater the number and the fewer the selection of tested relationships in a scientific field, the less likely the research findings are to be true.
4. The greater the flexibility in designs, definitions, outcomes, and analytical modes in a scientific field, the less likely the research findings are to be true.
5. The greater the financial and other interests and prejudices in a scientific field, the less likely the research findings are to be true.

6. The hotter a scientific field (the more scientific teams involved), the less likely the research findings are to be true.

Ioannides [7] then performs a pile of calculations and simulations but then demonstrates the likelihood of us getting at the truth from different typical study types (Table 1.1). This ranges from odds of 2:1 on (67% likely to be true) from a systematic review of good quality randomised trials, to 1:3 against (25% likely to be true) from a systematic review of small inconclusive randomised trials, to even lower levels for other architectures.

There is much more in these fascinating papers, but from here on in it all gets more detailed and more complex without becoming necessarily much easier to understand. There is nothing here that contradicts what we already know, namely that if we accept evidence of poor quality, without validity, or where there are few events or numbers of patients, we are likely, often highly likely, to be misled.

If we concentrate on evidence of high quality, which is valid, and with large numbers, that will hardly ever happen. As Ioannidis also comments, if instead of chasing some ephemeral statistical significance we concentrate our efforts where there is good prior evidence, our chances of getting the true result are better - concentrating on all the evidence. Which may be why clinical trials on pharmaceuticals are so often significant statistically, and in the direction of supporting a drug.

Yet even in that very special circumstance, where so much treasure is expended, years of work with positive results can come to naught when the big trials are done and do not produce the expected answer.

TABLE 1.1: LIKELIHOOD OF TRUTH OF RESEARCH FINDINGS FROM VARIOUS TYPICAL STUDY ARCHITECTURES

| Example | Ratio of true to not true |
| --- | --- |
| Confirmatory meta-analysis of good quality RCTs | 2:1 |
| Adequately powered RCT with little bias and 1:1 pre-study odds | 1:1 |
| Meta-analysis of small, inconclusive studies | 1:3 |
| Underpowered, but poorly performed phase I/II RCT | 1:5 |
| Underpowered, but well performed phase I/II RCT | 1:5 |
| Adequately powered exploratory epidemiological study | 1:10 |
| Underpowered exploratory epidemiological study | 1:10 |
| Discovery-orientated exploratory research with massive testing | 1:1,000 |

*"If a little knowledge is dangerous, where is the man who has so much as to be out of danger?"* (TH Huxley, 1877).

To avoid any hubris, it is always a good idea to acknowledge both the limitations of one's own knowledge, and that the constraint of writing with a particular voice can occasionally lead to flirtation with oversimplification. The aim is to help people overcome their concerns, and to help any consumer of evidence to feel comfortable with thinking about it. Many professionals, and members of the public, have helped Bandolier over the years by suggesting ways we could do things better, and being forthright about ways in which they would like data presented. A big thanks to all of them.

REFERENCES:

1.   R Smith, quoting Professor David Eddy, BMJ 1991 303: 798-799.
2.   LA Smith, AD Oldman, HJ McQuay, RA Moore. Teasing apart quality and validity in systematic reviews: an example from acupuncture trials in chronic neck and back pain. Pain 2000 86: 119-132.
3.   PM Rothwell, CN Martyn. Reproducibility of peer review in clinical neuroscience. Is agreement between reviewers any greater than would be expected by chance alone? Brain 2000 123: 1964-1969.
4.   M Bennett, R Heard. Treatment of multiple sclerosis with hyperbaric oxygen therapy. Undersea & Hyperbaric Medicine 2001 28: 117-122.
5.   M Deveugele et al. Consultation length in general practice: cross sectional study in six European countries BMJ 2002 325: 472-475.
6.   JPA Ioannides. Contradicted and initially stronger effects in highly cited clinical research. JAMA 2005 294: 218-228.
7.   JPA Ioannides. Why most published research findings are false. PLoS Medicine 2005 2: e124. (www.plosmedicine.org)

# Section 2

# Understanding clinical trial evidence

This section is about understanding evidence from clinical trials, which all comes down to understanding issues around quality, validity, and size, together with a minimal familiarity with the way in which results are reported. Interested readers will find more detail in Bandolier's Little Book of Understanding Evidence (Oxford University Press, 2006).

## Clinical trial fundamentals

While there are some fundamental properties necessary to produce a good clinical trial, what makes a clinical trial good depends on a number of factors. And there are different reasons for doing clinical trials – for instance proving whether one treatment is better than another requires a different approach from telling whether two treatments have the same effect. But we can make some important general observations about what to look for in a good clinical trial, and we know that if clinical trials of efficacy are not done properly, any results they produce will be worthless.

### Randomisation

We randomise trials to exclude selection bias. Trials are usually performed where there is uncertainty as to whether a treatment works (is better than no treatment or placebo), or whether one treatment is better than another. We start from a position of intellectual equipoise, that there is no proven difference between treatments. Trials are often done by believers, and belief, even subconscious belief, might influence choice of treatment for particular patients. To avoid this, and to ensure that the patients allocated to each intervention are as closely matched as possible, we make the treatment choice randomly. This might be by tossing a coin, or more often by computer-generated randomisation. If we do not randomise we can end up with treatment groups that are not the same, thus invalidating the trial, or with a trial that no-one will believe because trials that are not randomised are often shown to be wrong. Randomisation is essential.

Another important aspect of randomisation is concealment – hiding the result of random allocation from everyone involved in the trial. Concealment might be achieved by putting the treatment choice in a sealed envelope, for instance. That way no one can know in advance which treatment the next patient will have, and this again prevents patients being consciously or unconsciously selected for a particular treatment. Faulty methods of randomisation include assignment by date of birth, or hospital number, because they are not random (and treatment allocation may or may not be concealed).

Randomisation is important because we know that non-randomised or inadequately randomised studies tend to give over-optimistic results compared with those that are properly randomised (Table 2.1).

If a trial says it is properly randomised, how can we tell that it has been? The obvious thing is to look for a table describing the randomised groups of patients at the start of the trial. If randomisation has been done properly, the two groups should be very similar or identical to one another. So you would expect to see that average age, and age range, are about the same, with the same proportions of men and women, or patients with different severities of disease, or co-morbidities, or already being treated with certain therapies for those co-morbidities.

TABLE 2.1: BIAS IN CLINICAL TRIALS

| Feature | Overestimation of treatment effect |
| --- | --- |
| Trials not randomised | 40% |
| Trials not double-blind | 17% |
| Duplicate information | 20% |
| Small trials | 30% |
| Low reporting quality | 25% |

If trials are small (a few tens of patients), randomisation can fail because of the random play of chance. In reasonably sized trials with many tens or hundreds of patients, major discrepancy in patient characteristics implies that researchers have been very unlucky, or that there was a systematic failure in randomisation. Whether it is bad luck or failure to randomise properly, important differences between groups at the start of a trial are a good reason to be cautious about the result. In any event, it is worth checking any paper that describes itself as randomised, because some that do are not.

BLINDING

We conduct trials blind to minimise observer bias. Double blind means that neither the patient nor the healthcare professional knows which treatment has been given. Single blind means that the patient doesn't know but the healthcare professional does, or sometimes that the patient does but the healthcare professional making outcome assessments doesn't. It's belief again, because even if the trial is randomised, if we know that Mrs Jones has treatment A and Mr Smith treatment B, our observations may be biased by our belief that Mr Smith overstates his complaint and Mrs Jones understates hers. Only if we have no idea which treatment they received will we be free from a bias that is known to deliver incorrect results.

A good example of this is acupuncture for back pain [1]. Here the overall result was statistically in favour of acupuncture over the control, in this case a form of sham acupuncture, with acupuncture and control techniques checked by a panel of acupuncture experts. Yet as Figure 2.1 shows, those trials that were blind, where observers did not know what treatment patients had, showed negligible difference. Any difference came from trials in which the observers knew whether the patients had real acupuncture or sham acupuncture. Our conclusion might be that the best trials showed no effect, yet this meta-analysis has been used to demonstrate both that acupuncture is effective, and that it should be used to treat patients with back pain.

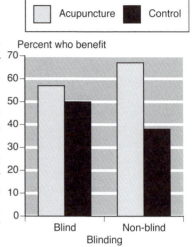

How do you know a trial has been properly blinded? The obvious thing is to look at the description of treatments used. If, for instance, they describe treatments as identical numbers of tablets, identical in appearance and taste, given at the same intervals during the day, that pretty much describes adequate double blinding, where neither patient nor professional should know who gets what. If there are different treatment regimens, then double-dummy techniques can be used. This might involve two sets of therapies, active A plus placebo B, or placebo A plus active B, and that can work for tablets or combinations of tablets and injection.

Sometimes blinding needs to be complicated. Homeopathy is often said to require individualisation for patients, a technique that is hard to blind. One method used an individualised homeopathic remedy as prescribed by a practitioner or placebo dispensed from a notary public, who held the randomisation schedule and mailed out the treatments. Reporting was to a study secretariat unconnected with the patients [2]. This was described as triple-blind.

Blinding is possible even for complicated interventions like surgery or homeopathy. Even so, it is worth checking the methods section of any paper that describes itself as double blind, because some trials that so describe themselves are not really double blind.

OTHER SOURCES OF BIAS

As Table 2.1 suggests, there are several other possible sources of bias. We know that study reports can be duplicated, sometimes in papers with completely different authors, but only the ones showing benefit. This can suggest there is a bigger literature of trials showing benefit than there actually is. Small trials, and those of poor reporting quality, also give better results than larger trials, and those of good reporting quality.

Bias is all in one direction, to produce better results. About 16-20 different sources of bias have been identified, and it is sometimes hard to keep track of them all. One that is worth bearing in mind is the issue of what happened to all the patients? Suppose 100 patients are randomised and enter a trial, but results are only reported on 50 of them because the other 50 dropped out or withdrew from treatment (a per-protocol analysis). What happened to the other 50 patients? Did they withdraw because of lack of efficacy, or because of adverse effects? Were there different reasons for withdrawal for treatment and control? If results are not reported and analysed according to all patients who entered the study, called intention to treat analysis, then bias may occur because we only see results in patients in whom the treatment worked or was tolerated.

## Placebo

Clinical trials sometimes, but not always, and in some cases never, compare treatment directly with placebo. The reason for using a placebo is that there are many circumstances where people get better by themselves, without intervention, or despite it. It is said that the common cold takes seven days to get better if you do nothing, but only one week if you treat it. In the example of back pain above, about 50-60% of patients had a "cure" when no active treatment was used, mostly in short term trials. That is exactly what we expect with back pain. If we did not have a placebo control, we might have thought that acupuncture was as miraculous as some enthusiasts claim. In other circumstances, like oncology, placebo on its own is almost never used, and instead we use add-on trials, where new treatments or placebo are compared when added on to treatments known to be effective.

Placebo deserves a section all on its own, to think about both how it is best used in clinical trials, and whether there is such a thing as the "placebo effect", where giving placebo has added benefit compared with doing nothing.

### Placebo response or placebo effect

This is perhaps one of the most difficult of all topics, especially with subjective outcomes such as pain or depression. If we were discussing a topic like myocardial infarction and our outcome measure was death, then we might be reasonably sure that a placebo would have no effect on the outcome. But with subjective outcomes like pain, or even erectile

Table 2.2: Possible effects of different types of control

| Control | Effects |
| --- | --- |
| Waiting list | Natural course of disease **minus** the negativity from nothing being done |
| Visits without treatment | Natural course of disease **plus** doctor/nurse/patient interaction |
| Placebo | Natural course of disease **plus** interaction **plus** expectation that there will be an effect |
| Active control | Natural course of disease **plus** interaction **plus** expectation **plus** actual effect |

dysfunction which can sometimes be psychogenic, we might guess that patients would feel better after placebo, and consequently have less pain or better erectile function, if the doctor or nurse was nice to them, or appeared authoritative, or if the placebo was given as a big red capsule instead of a tiny white pill, or as an injection and not a tablet. Whatever we think, proving that any or all of these influences had an effect would be difficult because very large trials would be necessary to show any effect independent of random chance. Table 2.2 summarises effects that we might expect to find in different control groups.

It is all very complicated, and made more so by the difficulty in proving that "negativity", or "interaction", or "expectation" contribute anything at all to the actual perception of benefit as it is measured. We don't help ourselves by using lax, if understandable, shorthand. When we want to discuss the effect that we observe when patients are given a placebo, we call it the "placebo effect" or placebo response. Immediately that can be retranslated as "the effect caused by placebo". Indirectly, of course, administration of placebo can and does result in an effect, for instance resulting in analgesia in a pain study. The pitfall is that we jump to a simplistic causal connection, and then in turn jump to conclusions about the mechanism by which this happens.

In erectile dysfunction trials variability in the response to placebo is rarely a problem, because there are only small differences between different PDE-5 inhibitors for some adverse event reporting [3], which were lower with sildenafil than tadalafil or vardenafil. This might simply reflect different expectations over time: when there is no effective treatment the attitude of a patient may be different from when there were known to be effective treatments.

## Validity

What constitutes trial validity is a difficult concept. The dictionary definition of valid is that which is sound or defensible, or having a premise from which the conclusion follows logically. We know it when we see it, or more particularly when our eyes are opened to its absence. Validity is always situation dependent, but criteria might include severity of illness at the start of a trial, the dose or intensity of the intervention, the duration of the intervention or the duration of observation.

For trials of erectile dysfunction, assessment of validity should be relatively simple. First is the issue of diagnosis – essentially how to measure erectile function. We now have the International Index of Erectile Function, discussed later, and several global measures that boil down to firm erections, adequate for penetration and successful intercourse. The second issue is one of setting: therapy, and trials, have to be in the domestic, not laboratory setting.

# Size

"There is much luck in the world, but it is luck. We are none of us safe". So said EM Forster nearly 100 years ago. It is astonishing how many people appreciate the importance of chance, in, say, winning a lottery or avoiding a car accident, but not in clinical trials. Perhaps it is all down to the way statistics are taught. We should forget probabilities and p-values, and acquaint ourselves with more relevant information, notably how much data we need to be sure that an observation is not likely to occur just by chance.

Why are people impressed with p-values? The cherished value of 0.05 merely says that a result is likely to have occurred by chance no more than 1 time in 20. Most of us have played Monopoly or other games involved with throwing dice. We will have experienced that throwing two sixes with two dice happens relatively often, yet the chance of that is about 1 time in 36.

Look at it another way. If you were about to cross a bridge, and were told that there was a 1 in 20 chance of it falling down when you were on it, would you take the chance? What about 1 in 100, or 1 in 1000? That p-value of 0.05 also tells you that 1 time in 20 the bridge is likely to fall down.

The dice analogy is pertinent, because there are now (at least) two papers that look at random chance and clinical trials, reminding us how often and how much chance can affect results. An older study actually used dice to mimic clinical trials in stroke prevention [4], while a second [5] used computer simulations of cancer therapy.

## DICE 1

In this study [4] participants in a practical class on statistics at a stroke course were given dice and asked to roll them a specified number of times to represent the treatment group of a randomised trial of a "new" treatment for stroke. If a six was thrown, this was recorded as a death, with any other number a survival. The procedure was repeated for a control group of similar size. Group size ranged from 5 to 100 patients.

The paper gives the results of all 44 trials for 2,256 "patients". While the paper does many clever things, it is perhaps more instructive to look at the results of the 44 trials. Since each arm of the trial looks for the throwing of one

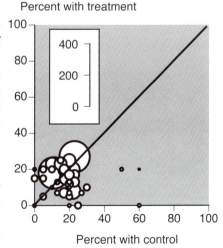

FIGURE 2.2: L'ABBÉ PLOT OF DICE 1 TRIALS

FIGURE 2.3: ODDS RATIOS FOR INDIVIDUAL DICE STUDIES, BY NUMBER IN "TRIAL". FILLED BARS WERE STATISTICALLY SIGNIFICANT

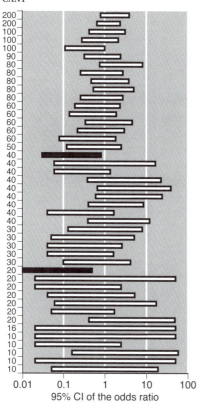

FIGURE 2.4: PERCENTAGE OF EVENTS IN EACH TRIAL ARM OF DICE "TRIALS"

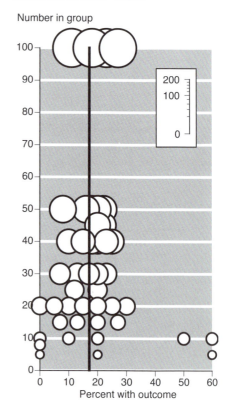

TABLE 2.3: META-ANALYSIS OF DICE TRIALS, WITH SENSITIVITY ANALYSIS BY SIZE OF TRIAL

| Analysis | Number of | | Outcome (%) wih | | Relative risk (95% CI) | NNT (95% CI) |
|---|---|---|---|---|---|---|
| | Trials | Patients | Treatment | Control | | |
| All trials | 44 | 2256 | 16.0 | 17.6 | 0.8 (0.5 to 1.1) | 62 (21 to -67) |
| Larger trials (>40 per group) | 11 | 1190 | 19.5 | 17.8 | 1.1 (0.9 to 1.4) | -60 (36 to -16) |
| Smaller trials (<40 per group) | 33 | 1066 | 12.0 | 17.3 | 0.7 (0.53 to 0.94) | 19 (11 to 98) |

out of six possibilities for standard dice, we might expect that the rate of events was 16.7% (100/6) in each, with an odds ratio or relative risk of 1.

Figure 2.2 shows a L'Abbé plot of the 44 trials. In a L'Abbé plot, each trial is represented by a symbol whose size is proportional to the size of the trial (shown by the inset scale); if there is no difference between treatments the symbols should fall along the line of equality. The expected result in this case is a grouping in the bottom left, on the line of equality, at about 17%. Actually, it is a bit more dispersed than that, with some trials far from the line of equality.

The odds ratios for individual trials are shown in Figure 2.3. Two trials (with 20 and 40 "patients" in total) had odds ratios statistically different from 1. That's one time in every 22 trials, and is what we expect by chance.

The variability in individual trial arms is shown in Figure 2.4, where the results are shown for all 88 of the trial arms. The vertical line shows the overall result, which was the 16.7% expected for 1 divided by 6. Larger samples come close to this, but small samples show values as low as zero, and as high as 60%.

The overall result, pooling data from all 44 trials, showed that events ("deaths") occurred in 16.0% of treatments and 17.6% of controls (overall mean 16.7%). The relative risk was 0.8 (0.5 to 1.1). The NNT was 62, with a 95% confidence interval that went from one benefit for every 21 treatments to one harm for every 67 treatments (Table 1.3.1).

Many of the experimental DICE trials were quite small, with as few as five per group. The smaller trials, with 40 per group or less, actually came up with a statistically significant result (Table 3). The NNT here was 19 (11 to 98).

## DICE 2

Information on the time between randomisation and death in a control group of 580 patients in a colorectal cancer trial was used to simulate 100 theoretical clinical trials. Each time the same 580 patients were randomly allocated to a theoretical treatment or control group, and survival curves calculated [5].

Four of the trials generated artificially had statistically significant results. One was significant at the p=0.003 level (1 in 333) and showed a large theoretical decrease in mortality of 40%.

Subgroup analysis was done for this trial by randomly allocating patients to group A or group B, and doing this 100 times. Over half (55%) of the subgroup analyses showed statistical significance between subgroups. The extremes of results were on the one hand no difference between subgroups, and on the other a result with a difference of very high statistically significance (0.00005, or 1 in 20,000). In another trial that had bare statistical significance, four of 100 simulated subgroups had statistical significance at the 1 in 100 level.

## WHAT DOES IT TELL US?

It emphasises that the random play of chance is a factor we cannot ignore, and that small trials are more prone to chance effects than larger ones. And it is not just an effect seen in single trials. Even when we pool data from small trials just from rolling dice, as in DICE 1, a meta-analysis can come up with a statistically significant effect when there was none.

High levels of statistical significance can be generated just by the random play of chance. DICE 2 found levels of statistical significance of 1 in 333 for at least one simulated trial, and 1 in 20,000 for a subgroup analysis of that trial.

Not only do we need well-conducted trials of robust design and reporting, we also need large amounts of information if the size of a clinical effect is to be assessed accurately. The rule of thumb is that where the difference between control and treatment is small we need very large amounts of information. Only when the difference is large (an absolute risk increase or decrease of 50%, affecting every second patient) can we be reasonably happy with information from 500 patients or less.

When we see differences in results between trials, or between responses to placebo, the rush is often to try and explain away the difference as due to some facet of trial design or patient characteristic. Almost never does anyone ask how likely it is that the difference occurred just by the random play of chance.

## How results are reported

Understanding clinical trials and systematic reviews and meta-analyses involves not just how trials are conducted and what constitutes a good or bad trial, but how to comprehend and use results from a trial. Any time we read a clinical trial report or a systematic review we need to think not about one or two factors, but many.

For instance, we tend to think of clinical trials as having numbers attached to them, measuring outcomes (reduction in cholesterol with statin) and statistical significance (a significant reduction in cholesterol with statin). When we analyse systematic reviews we have become accustomed to meta-analysis, where we do sums on clinical trials with numbers. This would be a quantitative review.

We can also do qualitative reviews, where it may have been impossible to pool results from different trials because, for instance, different outcomes were measured. What we might then do is to say that we have trials measuring different things, but they all showed a statistically significant benefit in the different things measured. In qualitative reviews we end up vote counting, in which each trial has one "vote". We count up positives, negatives, and neutrals. The problem with this is that one large, well-conducted trial can be outvoted by more small, poorly conducted trials. Vote counting can lead us astray because it takes no account of either the size of the trial or the size of the treatment effect in a trial.

For quantitative reviews, even if trials and review are impeccably conducted, we have to get our heads around how the results are described. This can be not just in one way but many, often statistical. We have to comprehend the results before we can use them, and how those results are reported affects our comprehension.

There is probably no single "best" way of reporting results so that everyone will comprehend them. We are all very different in our tastes. It is not surprising that we vary in the facility with which our minds grasp and manipulate different concepts. Some of us will be happiest with complex statistical concepts. Others, and Bandolier is one of those, are happiest with the simplest representations.

## The meaning of words

**Output** - "quantity produced or turned out; data after processing by a computer". This dictionary definition differentiates between two different and important qualities of results of clinical trials. One, and perhaps that most useful to practitioners, is the quantity of benefit or harm a treatment is going to produce in patients like those in the trial or review. If it were a car, it would be equivalent to how fast it would go, or the fuel economy. The other is a statistical result, often a comparison with some other intervention, perhaps placebo. Again, if it were a car, this would tell us whether this car went faster than another car, or had better or worse fuel efficiency.

But we can drive only one car at a time. It might be nice to know that my car is more fuel efficient than yours, but it is the car I am driving, and I want to know how many litres per 100 kilometres, or miles per gallon, my car does, because otherwise I might run out of petrol. If our best evidence comes from randomised trials and systematic reviews, then one of the most important things is how that trial or review gives us the result. From a clinical point of view we want to know how much benefit (or harm) a treatment will produce, and results of data processing might not be much help.

**Utility** - "usefulness: the power to satisfy the wants of people in general". If systematic reviews are to be useful, and therefore used, they have to present results in ways that are immediately accessible to ordinary professionals. Rapid understanding is important for busy people. Trying to work out what a hazard ratio or an effect size means to treating the patient in front of us will not make for an easy morning surgery.

TABLE 2.4: HYPOTHETICAL ACUTE PAIN TRIAL: EER IS EXPERIMENTAL EVENT RATE, CER IS CONTROL EVENT RATE, AND NNT IS NUMBER NEEDED TO TREAT

| Treatment | Total number of patients treated | Number achieving at least 50% pain relief | Number not achieving at least 50% pain relief |
|---|---|---|---|
| Ibuprofen 400 mg | 40 | 22 | 18 |
| Placebo | 40 | 7 | 33 |

**Calculations made from these results**

| | |
|---|---|
| Experimental event rate (EER, event rate with ibuprofen) | 22/40 = 0.55 or 55% |
| Control event rate (CER, event rate with placebo) | 7/40 = 0.18 or 18% |
| Experimental event odds | 22/18 = 1.2 |
| Control event odds | 7/33 = 0.21 |
| Odds ratio | 1.2/0.21 = 5.7 |
| Relative risk (EER/CER) | 0.55/0.18 =3.1 |
| Relative risk increase (100(EER-CER)/CER )) as a percentage | 100((0.55-0.18)/0.18) = 206% |
| Absolute risk increase or reduction (EER-CER) | 0.55 - 0.18 = 0.37 (or 37%) |
| NNT (1/(EER-CER)) | 1/(0.55 - 0.18) = 2.7 |

DEFINING OUTPUTS

Most of the outputs that we use for reporting trials and reviews have their origins in epidemiology, the world where we look for small effects in large populations – things like aspirin after a heart attack, or reducing cholesterol. Most of the activity of medicine is, conversely, about large effects in small populations, like hip replacements for osteoarthritic joints, or pain relief for migraine, or antibiotics for infection.

Table 2.4 is a hypothetical trial of ibuprofen in acute pain. Not worrying too much at this stage about any other features or even the result itself, we will use this trial to give definitions of some of the more common outputs where information is available  in dichotomous form. Dichotomous means the patient had the outcome or did not, and we have the numbers for each. In this trial, for instance, 22 of 40 patients given ibuprofen had adequate pain relief compared with only 7 of 40 given placebo. The term experimental event rate (EER) is used to describe the rate at which good events occur with ibuprofen (22/40, or 55%) and control event rate (CER) to describe the rate at which good events occur with placebo (7/40 or 18%).

| Event rates | | | |
|---|---|---|---|
| Experimental | Control | Odds ratio | Relative risk |
| 3 | 1 | 2.8 | 3.0 |
| 6 | 2 | 2.8 | 3.0 |
| 12 | 4 | 3.0 | 3.0 |
| 24 | 8 | 3.3 | 3.0 |
| 48 | 16 | 4.3 | 3.0 |
| 60 | 20 | 5.3 | 3.0 |
| 90 | 30 | 12.0 | 3.0 |

## ODDS RATIOS

This Table shows first how to compute odds. Odds refers to the ratio of the number of people *having* the good event to the number *not having* the good event, so the experimental event odds are 22/18 or 1.2. The odds ratio is the ratio of the odds with experimental treatment to that of control, or here 1.2/0.21 = 5.7. There are different ways of computing odds ratios that give slightly different answers in different circumstances. Values greater than 1 show that experimental is better than control, and if a 95% confidence interval is calculated, statistical significance is assumed if the interval does not include 1.

Some would change this around and compute the odds ratios from the point of view of the patients **not** having adequate pain relief. The experimental event odds would be 18/22 or 0.82, and the control event odds would be 33/7 or 4.7. The odds ratio then would be 0.82/4.7 = 0.17.

For ibuprofen versus placebo the odds ratio is 5.7 or 0.17. Pick the bones out of that. How would you use that, other than knowing that an odds ratio that was far from 1 meant that ibuprofen was better than placebo?

## RELATIVE RISK OR BENEFIT

Relative risk is a bit easier on the brain. It is simply the ratio of EER to CER, here 0.55/0.18 (or 55/18 for percentages), and is 3.1. Again values greater than 1 show that experimental is better than control, and if a 95% confidence interval is calculated, statistical significance is assumed if the interval does not include 1. Odds ratios and relative risk tend to concur when event rates are low, but not when event rates are high. Table 2.5 shows this for a series of hypothetical examples where the experimental event rate is always three times higher than the control event rate. The relative risk is always 3, but the odds ratio varies from 2.8 to 12. There is disagreement between eminent statisticians about which of these is "best". We (and Bandolier) use relative risk whenever possible, but wouldn't pick a fight with someone who preferred odds ratios.

Again, knowing that the relative risk is 3.1 is not intuitively useful. Both relative risk and odds ratio are important ways of ensuring that there is statistical significance in our result. Unless there is statistical significance, we should not be using a treatment except in exceptional circumstances. So whatever else we do in the way of data manipulation, statistical significance of one or other of these tests gives us the right to move on.

## Relative risk increase or reduction

The relative risk increase is the difference between the EER and CER (EER-CER) divided by the CER, and usually expressed as a percentage. In Table 2.4 the relative risk increase is 206%. If the number of events is smaller with treatment, then the relative risk reduction is calculated by subtracting the CER from EER in the equation.

## Absolute risk increase or reduction

If we subtract the CER from the EER (EER-CER) then we have the absolute risk increase (ARI), the effect due solely to the treatment, and nothing else. The language here doesn't quite work because it was originally taken from the world of epidemiology where reducing risk (cholesterol lowering etc) is all. The absolute risk reduction (ARR) is CER-EER, when events occur more often with control than they do with treatment.

## Number needed to treat (NNT)

For every 100 patients with acute pain treated with ibuprofen, 37 (= 55 - 18) will have adequate pain relief because of the ibuprofen we have given them. Clearly then, we have to treat 100/37, or 2.7 patients with ibuprofen for one to benefit because of the ibuprofen they have been given. That's what NNT is (Table 2.4). This has immediate clinical relevance because we immediately know what clinical and other effort is being made to produce one result with a particular intervention.

The best NNT would be 1, where everyone got better with treatment and nobody got better with control, and NNTs close to 1 can be found with antibiotic treatments for susceptible organisms, for instance. Higher NNTs represent less good treatment, and the NNT is a useful tool for comparing two similar treatments. When doing so the NNT must always specify the comparator (eg, placebo, no treatment, or some other treatment), the therapeutic outcome, and the duration of treatment necessary to achieve that outcome. If these are different, you probably should not be comparing NNTs. It is also worth mentioning that prophylactic interventions that produce small effects in large numbers of patients will have high NNTs, perhaps 20-100. Just because an NNT is large does not mean it will not be a useful preventive medicine.

## NUMBER NEEDED TO HARM (NNH)

We can use the same methods for adverse events, when numbers needed to treat become numbers needed to harm (NNH). Here small numbers are bad (more frequent harm) and larger numbers good. When making comparisons between treatments, the same provisos apply as for NNT, the need to specify the type of harm, the comparator, and the dose and duration of therapy.

For both NNT and NNH we should recognise that we are working with an unusual scale running from 1 (everyone has the intended outcome with treatment and none with control) to –1 (no-one has outcome with treatment and everyone has it with control), with infinity as the mid point where we divide by zero when experimental event rate equals control event rate. Once NNTs or NNHs are much above 10 the upper confidence interval gets closer to infinity and the upper and lower intervals look unbalanced.

## Comment

There's no single answer as to which output works best for everyone, or anyone, or for particular circumstances. Graphical representations may be better than numbers in aiding comprehension of clinical trial results. The main thing is to be sure that you know and understand whatever output you choose, and especially not to be swayed by things like relative risk, or odds ratios, or relative risk reduction, or whatever, when some of these can be highly statistically significant but clinically irrelevant.

Few clinical trials and few systematic reviews will give you results in the way that you want them, so there's no escaping doing some work yourself.

We have found it most useful to follow the following procedures when looking at outputs from systematic reviews and meta-analyses:

1. First check on the statistical result (relative risk or benefit, or odds ratio).
2. **IF** statistically significant, proceed to calculate an NNT. Use NNT to estimate the ***treatment specific therapeutic effort*** needed for one outcome, which puts some clinical relevance on the result.
3. **IF** this seems sensible, look at what percentage of patients benefit from (or are harmed by) treatment, and use this figure for every day work because this is immediately clinically relevant every time.

It seems to work, if only because we can remember and use percentages quite easily, and because that is what is relevant in everyday practice. The bottom line, though, is what people can use effectively in their day-to-day practice. Once statistics are done with, perhaps the best thing to remember, if there is only room for one number, is the percentage of people benefiting (or being harmed) by the treatment.

But statistics are less important than knowing that trials are performed properly. If trial design is inadequate, and allows bias to creep in, then statistics are useless. If trials are invalid, because they do not tell us what we want to know, then statistics are useless. If there are insufficient numbers of patients or events, then any result can be overwhelmed by the random play of chance, and, again, statistics are useless.

REFERENCES:

1. E Ernst, AR White. Acupuncture for back pain: A meta-analysis of randomised controlled trials. Archives of Internal Medicine 1998 158: 2235-2241.
2. H Walach et al. Classical homeopathic treatment of chronic headaches. Cephalalgia 1997 17: 119-126.
3. RA Moore et al. Indirect comparison of interventions using published randomised trials: Systematic review of PDE-5 inhibitors for erectile dysfunction. BMC Urology 2005 5: 18 (www.biomedcentral.com/1471-2490/5/18/abstract)
4. CE Counsell et al. The miracle of DICE therapy for acute stroke: fact or fictional product of subgroup analysis? BMJ 1994 309: 1677-1681.
5. M Clarke, J Halsey. DICE2: a further investigation of the effects of chance in life, death and subgroup analyses. International Journal of Clinical Practice 2001 55: 240-242.

# SECTION 3

# ERECTILE DYSFUNCTION TRIALS

Before even starting to perform trials, the most important thing is to establish what it is that is to be measured. For erectile dysfunction, the most important thing is erectile function, and when a new therapy is created in what is essentially a previously untreated condition, or one treated, but often ineffectively, new measurement tools have to be produced. This was the situation when sildenafil began to be tested in the 1990s.

The basic measurement tool used in the sildenafil studies was a self-administered measure of erectile dysfunction, the International Index of Erectile Function (IIEF) [1]. The importance of this instrument is that it was developed to examine the main features of erectile dysfunction, was quick and simple to complete, and had sensitivity and specificity to detect treatment-related changes in erectile dysfunction. It had 15 questions, easily scored, and was destined to be the core tool for a useful diagnostic aid in erectile dysfunction.

## Diagnostic tool for erectile function

The key features of the scale and its development were:

- It had 15 questions dealing with erectile function, orgasmic function, sexual desire, intercourse satisfaction and overall satisfaction.
- Based on literature search of existing questionnaires.
- Developed from an initial questionnaire after trials with patients and review by an expert panel.
- Validated in ten languages.
- Examined for validity in a number of contexts.

These criteria fulfilled most criteria for an evidence-based measurement instrument. The part of the full questionnaire most frequently used was the erectile function domain of five questions (Table 3.1). The 15 questions of the original IIEF have been examined for their usefulness as a simple patient-administered diagnostic tool of erectile dysfunction, using information gathered in randomised trials [2].

STUDY

In trials men had to be 18 or older, in a stable heterosexual relationship for at least six months and have a clinical diagnosis of erectile dysfunction. Erectile dysfunction was of organic, psychogenic or mixed aetiology, but anatomic disorders or patients with severe concomitant disease were excluded. A control group of men without a history of erectile dysfunction was recruited. There were 932 men with erectile dysfunction and 115 controls. Using baseline data from the randomised trials, items on the IIEF scale were examined for their ability to discriminate between men with and without erectile dysfunction.

TABLE 3.1: IIEF-5 SCORING SYSTEM

| Over the past six months: | | Score | | | |
|---|---|---|---|---|---|
| | 1 | 2 | 3 | 4 | 5 |
| How do you rate your confidence that you could get and keep an erection? | Very low | Low | Moderate | High | Very high |
| When you had erections with sexual stimulation, how often were your erections hard enough for penetration? | Almost never or never | Much less than half the time | About half the time | Much more than half the time | Almost always or always |
| During sexual intercourse, how often were you able to maintain your erection after you had penetrated (entered) your partner? | Almost never or never | Much less than half the time | About half the time | Much more than half the time | Almost always or always |
| During sexual intercourse how difficult was it to maintain your erection to the completion of intercourse? | Extremely difficult | Very difficult | Difficult | Slightly difficult | Not difficult |
| When you attempted sexual intercourse, how often was it satisfactory for you? | Almost never or never | Much less than half the time | About half the time | Much more than half the time | Almost always or always |

The IIEF-5 score is the sum of questions 1 to 5. The lowest score is 5 and the highest score 25.

Of the 15 questions, six had moderate or good discrimination between men with and without erectile dysfunction, while for nine it was very poor to the extent of being nonexistent. The ability to maintain erections during sexual intercourse was the best discriminator (100%).

Five questions were chosen (Table 3.1) in which the maximum score was 25 and the minimum 5. Men without erectile dysfunction had a mean score of 23 and men with erectile dysfunction had a mean score of 11. These were evaluated in a number of ways, but principally to define a cut point above which erectile dysfunction would be unlikely, and below which it would be likely.

That cut point was determined to be a score of 21. This score had a sensitivity of 98% and specificity of 88%, giving a likelihood ratio for a positive test of 8 and for a negative result of 0.02.

Let us assume that there is a 50% chance of men visiting their GP about erectile dysfunction truly suffering from it. If such a man scored 21 or less, then their chance of truly having erectile dysfunction rises to about 93%. If they score 22 or more, then it falls to 2% or less.

COMMENT ON DIAGNOSTIC TOOL

This is useful because of its simplicity, and because it can be used both in clinical trials and as a diagnostic tool for clinical practice. It provides us with a scale easily completed by patients, and from the final score an indication of severity. Scores of 22 or more indicate normality.

## Sildenafil trials

One systematic review of sildenafil trials [3] is helpful because it was conducted using clinical trial reports. These are detailed documents produced by pharmaceutical companies for internal and registration purposes. They are much more detailed than published papers, which are often limited to a few thousand words. By contrast, clinical trial reports can run to hundreds, even thousands, of pages, and provide in depth analysis, and are particularly useful for adverse event information, as well as describing efficacy in a number of different ways.

For the review, a prior definition of efficacy was a man with a consistent three-part outcome, consisting of an erection, sufficiently rigid for penetration, and followed by successful intercourse. Other efficacy outcomes of interest were the number of men with the highest two responses on the International Index of Erectile Function (IIEF) questions 3 and 4, and global evaluations of treatment efficacy by patients [9]. The number of grade 3 or 4 erections (at least hard enough for penetration) and successful erections were also noted.

Adverse events were also sought. These were the number of men with any treatment-related adverse event, the total number of men discontinuing, those discontinuing through lack of efficacy or through adverse events, adverse events rated severe or serious, and information on particular adverse events.

Outcomes actually available and chosen were:

### EFFICACY

- Number of men in whom the proportion of successful attempts at sexual intercourse was more than 60%
- Number of men in whom the proportion of successful attempts at sexual intercourse was more than 40%
- Number of men reporting that their erections had been improved on a global question ("Has the treatment you have been taking over the past four weeks improved your erections?").

### ERECTIONS

- The weighted mean number of weekly erections was calculated.
- The weighted mean success rate was calculated.
- The weighted mean weekly number of successful occasions where intercourse occurred was calculated from these numbers.

### ADVERSE EVENTS

- Treatment-related adverse events
- Severe adverse events
- Serious adverse events
- Dyspepsia
- Headache
- Vasodilation (flushing)

### DISCONTINUATIONS

- All-cause discontinuations
- Discontinuations due to inefficacy
- Discontinuations due to adverse events

## Dose

A prior intention in this review was to analyse effectiveness and harm according to dose. This is important, because benefit and harm from interventions is often dose dependent. In erectile function therapy, dosing can be fixed, or optimised, where men take an initial dose of 50 mg, and then move up to 100 mg or down to 25 mg on subsequent occasions depending on their individual judgement of the efficacy or any adverse events caused by that dose.

## Trials available

Twenty-seven clinical trial reports were made available, all prepared for a marketing authorisation application, and dated before September 1997. Some of these were single dose use in laboratory setting with penile plethysmography as an outcome. Others were open extensions of randomised studies. These were not useful, and 17 were excluded. All ten of the included clinical trial reports had a quality score of 3 (two) or 4 (eight) out of a maximum of 5 on a standard quality of reporting scale. All were randomised but only two stated how randomisation was achieved. All stated that they were double blind, and six explained how blinding was achieved (double-dummy, identical placebo). All studies described withdrawals clearly and were performed on an intention-to-treat basis incorporating patients with unsuccessful attempts for reasons not associated with sildenafil.

## Typical patients

For inclusion in a study a man had to have a minimum six-month history of erectile dysfunction, be 18 years or older, be in a heterosexual relationship for at least six months and be able to give written consent. There was typically a long (21 point) list of exclusions that included anatomical deformities, other sexual disorders, diabetes with poor control and/or untreated proliferative retinopathy, recent (six month) history of heart attack or stroke, significant cardiovascular disease, active peptic ulceration or bleeding, use of other treatments for erectile dysfunction and known history of retinitis pigmentosa.

All of the clinical exclusions were sensible and would form part of clinical advice regarding advisability of starting this treatment outside a trial. Nine of the ten studies described men as having erectile dysfunction of organic, mixed or psychogenic aetiology; a small number of men in the trials also had diabetes.

Typically men would attend for a screening visit to record medical information and to have a physical examination. Treatments were to be taken as required before anticipated sexual activity on an outpatient basis over periods up to 12 weeks. No more than one treatment was to be taken on any one day.

**FIGURE 3.1:** IMPROVED ERECTIONS AND ADVERSE EVENTS WITH DIFFERENT FIXED DOSE AND DOSE OPTIMISED SILDENAFIL SCHEDULES

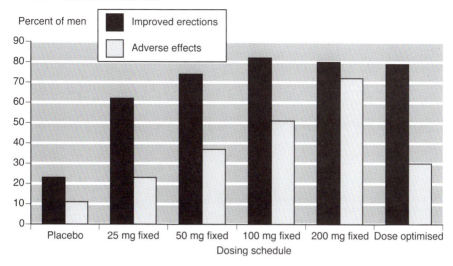

**FIGURE 3.2:** MEAN NUMBER OF ERECTIONS A WEEK AND THE NUMBER OF ERECTIONS RESULTING IN SUCCESSFUL INTERCOURSE

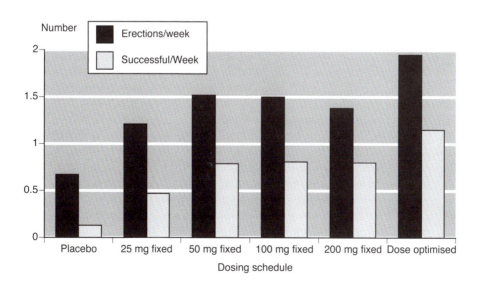

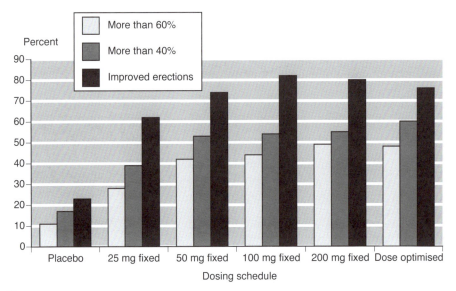

FIGURE 3.3: MEAN PERCENTAGE OF MEN ACHIEVING THE EFFICACY OUTCOMES

## RESULTS

The main results of a larger meta-analysis with more men are reported in a later section. The point here is to comment upon the types of results which can be obtained from trials, at least when the full details of clinical trial reports are available. A number of study descriptions were possible from clinical trial reports which would be unlikely to be reported in published versions of the same studies, because of lack of space.

For instance, Figure 3.1 shows the effect of dose on improved erections, and on men reporting at least one adverse event. There is a clear, but different, dose response for efficacy and harm using fixed dosing schedules. There is a better profile, maximising benefit and minimising harm, using an adjusted dose schedule.

Moreover, different outcomes from the same trials can be compared. Figure 3.2 gives information on the number of erections men had each week, and the number of times they had successful intercourse (consisting of an erection, sufficiently rigid for penetration, and followed by successful intercourse). Figure 3.3 shows the percentage of men who had successful intercourse more than 40% of the time, more than 60% of the time, and who just had improved erections.

Results like this cannot be obtained from published clinical trials, yet the information is almost certainly contained within the clinical trial reports. Important information, especially about potentially useful outcomes of trials, is lost by not using clinical trial reports.

| Studies | Incidence (Percent and 95% CI) | |
| --- | --- | --- |
| | Placebo | Sildenafil |
| **Phase II/III placebo-controlled** | | |
| Serious cardiovascular events | 5.7 (3.3 to 8.2) | 4.1 (2.7 to 5.5) |
| Myocardial infarction | 1.4 (0.2 to 2.6) | 1.7 (0.8 to 2.6) |
| **Phase II/III open-label extensions** | | |
| Serious cardiovascular events | | 3.5 (2.3 to 4.7) |
| Myocardial infarction | | 1.0 (0.3 to 1.6) |

Serious cardiovascular events include myocardial infarction, angina and coronary artery disorders

RARE ADVERSE EVENTS

However good clinical trials may be, a more complete analysis from several trials is probably needed to pick up rare but serious adverse events. Because the men who will be prescribed sildenafil will have cardiovascular risk factors, like hypertension, hyperlipidaemia and diabetes, any effect on cardiovascular events is very important.

An analysis of all 18 placebo-controlled trials [4] showed no difference in the incidence of myocardial infarction, angina or coronary artery disorders between sildenafil use and placebo (4274 men), nor was the incidence higher in the 2199 men taking part in open label extensions (Table 3.2). Blood pressure and heart rate were unaffected.

## Comment

What we have is the development of trial methods in a new area. The criteria used in the trials were good, and the reporting, at least in clinical trial reports, excellent. Serious but rare adverse events have been looked for. Because erectile dysfunction is a new area, investigated in an era when we have been concerned with possible sources of bias, the trials themselves conformed to good practice, and have been properly randomised, and properly blind, and tell us about the fate of each individual. In the area of PDE-5 inhibitors, we have a body of information which is difficult to fault, except in the one area of reporting of outcomes. Too many published papers are unable to provide the information we really want, which is the triple outcome consisting of an erection, sufficiently rigid for penetration, and followed by successful intercourse.

REFERENCES:

1   RC Rosen et al. The international index of erectile dysfunction (IIEF): a multidimensional scale for assessment of erectile dysfunction. Urology 1997 49: 822-830.
2   RC Rosen et al. Development and evaluation of an abridged, 5-item version of the international index of erectile function (IIEF-5) as a diagnostic tool for erectile dysfunction. International Journal of Impotence Research 1999 11: 319-326.
3   RA Moore et al. Sildenafil (Viagra) for male erectile dysfunction: a meta-analysis of clinical trial reports. BMC Urology 2002 2:6. (http://www.biomedcentral.com/1471-2490/2/6/).
4   A Morales et al. Clinical safety of oral sildenafil citrate (VIAGRA) in the treatment of erectile dysfunction. International Journal of Impotence Research 1998 10: 69-74.

# SECTION 4

# COMMON SEXUAL PROBLEMS IN WOMEN AND MEN

# Sexual dysfunction survey in the USA

## Clinical bottom line

Sexual problems are common for adults, both on a lifetime basis and on a current basis. Many respondents would choose help from their family doctor.

As medicine and lifestyle become inextricably mixed, dealing with issues concerning sexual dysfunction is more common. The increase of interest in male erectile problems is just one part of this, so any study which sheds more light on just how common problems are is helpful.

## Study

As part of a US National Health and Social Life Survey, questions were asked of men and women aged between 18 and 59 years [1]. There were 1410 men and 1749 women, with exclusions of people living in group quarters (barracks, dormitories, prisons) and people not fluent in English. Seventy-nine percent of people asked took part in the survey.

## Results

The answers for six questions given to both men and women are shown in Table 4.1.

For most questions there was little difference in response rates with age, except pain during sex (higher in the youngest age group of women), sex not pleasurable (lowest in the oldest age group of women), and trouble achieving or maintaining an erection (increased with age in men, Figure 4.1).

Clearly there was a high overall rate of problems, with 32% of women lacking interest in sex, 26% unable to achieve orgasm and 16% experiencing pain during sex. For men, early climax and anxiety about per-

TABLE 4.1: COMMON SEXUAL PROBLEMS IN WOMEN AND MEN

| Question | Percent |
|---|---|
| **Women** | |
| Lack interest in sex | 32 |
| Unable to achieve orgasm | 26 |
| Experience pain during sex | 16 |
| Sex not pleasurable | 23 |
| Anxious about performance | 12 |
| Trouble lubricating | 21 |
| **Men** | |
| Lack interest in sex | 15 |
| Unable to achieve orgasm | 8 |
| Climax too early | 31 |
| Sex not pleasurable | 8 |
| Anxious about performance | 18 |
| Trouble achieving or maintaining erection | 10 |

formance were major problems, but in the age group of 50-59 years 18% had trouble achieving or maintaining an erection.

The study also showed that the experience of sexual dysfunction is highly associated with unsatisfying personal experiences and relationships. There were strong (and probably causal) relationships between low sexual desire or performance with low physical and emotional satisfaction and low general happiness.

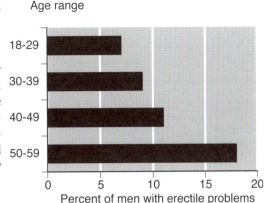

FIGURE **4.1:** MEN WITH ERECTILE PROBLEMS, BY AGE

## COMMENT

When clever chemists, by chance or design, develop safe and effective drugs which help women achieve an orgasm, or which relieve pain during sex, then there will be a stampede to obtain those drugs, just as there has been for effective treatments for male erectile dysfunction. For many people poor sexual life translates into lower general happiness.

Given that most people recognise that life is not a rehearsal, but the real thing, and that sexual problems are common, then you don't have to be a rocket scientist to see this as a major growth area. In the UK, and probably in other countries, some imaginative solutions will be needed to how we deal with lifestyle, health and medical resources.

REFERENCE:

1    EO Laumann, A Paik, RC Rosen. Sexual dysfunction in the United States: prevalence and predictors. JAMA 1999 281: 537-544.

# Sexual health survey in the UK

## Clinical bottom line

Sexual problems are common for UK adults, both on a lifetime basis and on a current basis. Many respondents would choose help from their family doctor.

---

## Survey [1]

Four diverse general practices in England participated, and from each register a random sample of 1000 people was selected of men and women in different age groups between the ages of 18 and 75. A questionnaire was piloted and then sent to the selected individuals from the registers, with a letter from the practice emphasising the importance of the work and the anonymity of the questionnaire. Questionnaires for men and women were different.

## Results

The response rate was 39% for men and 49% for women, with 1768 responses in total. One third of responders had not had sex at all during the previous three months, and one fifth reported having sex more than once a week.

The current and lifetime sexual problems reported by women and men are shown in Table 4.2. For women, vaginal dryness and never or rarely experiencing a climax were common. For men common problems were getting and maintaining an erection, and premature ejaculation.

About half the responders said they would like to receive help for sexual problems, but only about 5% of those who wanted help had received it.

Given an opportunity to choose whence such help would be most welcome, there

TABLE 4.2: Common sexual problems in women and men in the UK

| Problem | Percent with sexual problem | |
|---|---|---|
| | Current | Lifetime |
| **Women** | | |
| Never or rarely climax | 27 | |
| Pain during intercourse | 18 | 45 |
| Vaginal dryness | 28 | 49 |
| Problems with arousal | 17 | |
| Sex never or rarely pleasant | 18 | |
| **Any of these** | 41 | |
| **Any lifetime problem** | | 68 |
| **Men** | | |
| Difficulty getting erection | 21 | 23 |
| Difficulty maintaining erection | 24 | 25 |
| Either or both of these | 26 | 39 |
| Premature ejaculation | 14 | 31 |
| Sex never or rarely pleasant | 9 | |
| **Any of these** | 34 | |
| **Any lifetime problem** | | 54 |

was a preference for family doctor, family planning or well (wo)man clinic or trained marriage guidance counsellor.

COMMENT

These results are strikingly similar to those found in the US survey. It highlights a high prevalence of sexual problems, with a gap between need and provision. As always with this type of problem and survey, there are elements of medical problems, and of social problems, and both will vary depending on circumstances. What this sort of survey provides, though, is a useful insight into issues likely to come to the fore in the future.

REFERENCE:

1    KM Dunn, PR Croft, GI Hackett. Sexual problems: a study of the prevalence and need for health care in the general population. Family Practice 1998 15: 519-524.

# WORLDWIDE SURVEY OF ATTITUDES TO SEX AND PROBLEMS IN WOMEN AND MEN

## CLINICAL BOTTOM LINE

Sexual problems for older adults differ in different parts of the world. About four in ten women and three in ten men aged 40-80 years has at least one problem related to sex or intercourse.

---

A number of studies in different parts of the world have examined various aspects of male and female sexual attitudes and dysfunction. This very large study took a global perspective.

## STUDY

This was a very large study in several parts of the world, including:

- Northern Europe: Austria, Belgium, Germany, Sweden, UK
- Southern Europe: France, Israel, Italy, Spain
- Non-European West: Australia, Canada, NZ, South Africa, USA
- Central/South America: Brazil, Mexico
- Middle East: Algeria, Egypt, Morocco, Turkey
- East Asia: China, HK, Japan, Korea, Taiwan
- South East Asia: Indonesia, Malaysia, Philippines, Singapore, Thailand

A random selection of adults aged 40 to 80 years was selected, and various methods used for a questionnaire survey, using same-gender interviewers. Questions related to demographics, health, relationships, sexual behaviour, and beliefs.

Respondents were asked specific questions about one or more sexual problems occurring for two months or more during the previous year. Those responding sometimes or frequently were rated as having the problem.

## RESULTS

The final total of 27,516 respondents was 19% of the initial eligible population. The average age was 53-57 years, and 70-90% of adults were married or in an ongoing relationship. About 70% reported excellent health, though the figure was only about 50% for Middle-eastern and South-Asian women, and women generally reported somewhat worse health than men. Between 20% and 35% reported hypertension and 8-17% diabetes.

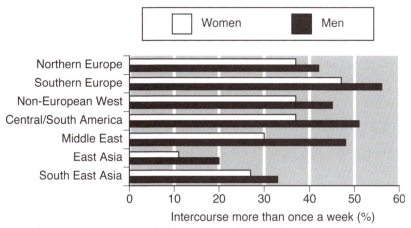

Consistently more men (75-90%) than women (50-70%) reported intercourse in the last 12 months. Intercourse frequency of more than once a week was highly variable (Figure 4.2).

FEMALE SEXUAL DYSFUNCTION

Four in 10 women aged 40-80 years had at least one problem (Table 4.3), with lack of interest in sex the most frequent. There were quite large differences between regions, with lowest rates in Northern Europe (Figure 4.3).

TABLE 4.3: PREVALENCE OF SEXUAL DYSFUNCTIONS IN WOMEN, TOTAL COHORT

| Problem | Percent with problem |
|---|---|
| Lack of interest in sex | 21 |
| Inability to achieve orgasm | 16 |
| Lubrication difficulties | 16 |
| Sex not pleasurable | 15 |
| Pain during sexual intercourse | 10 |
| At least one problem | 39 |

Denominator is the number of women with at least one sexual encounter in the previous 12 months

TABLE 4.4: PREVALENCE OF SEXUAL DYSFUNCTIONS IN MEN, TOTAL COHORT

| Problem | Percent with problem |
|---|---|
| Early ejaculation | 14 |
| Erection difficulty | 10 |
| Lack of interest in sex | 9 |
| Inability to achieve orgasm | 7 |
| Sex not pleasurable | 6 |
| At least one problem | 28 |

Denominator is the number of men with at least one sexual encounter in the previous 12 months

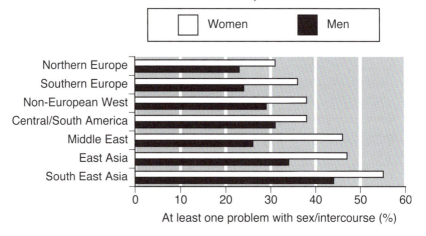

## MALE SEXUAL DYSFUNCTION

Three in 10 men aged 40-80 years had at least one problem (Table 4.4), with early ejaculation the most frequent. There were quite large differences between regions, with lowest rates in Northern Europe (Figure 4.3).

## COMMENT

Additional analysis by age and frequency of problems showed, as expected, that frequent problems are found more often at older age. For women there was a shallow relationship between problems and age, while for men there was a strong relationship with age for erectile difficulties, lack of sexual interest, and inability to reach orgasm. The results from this large worldwide study confirm results previously seen in the USA and UK.

These surveys all look at the prevalence of sexual problems in the general population. Clearly higher rates of erectile problems will occur in men with particular clinical conditions, like diabetes or heart disease.

Other publications from the survey did not show any more consistent relationships between sexual problems and demographic factors.

## REFERENCE:

1   A Nicolosi et al. Sexual behaviour and sexual dysfunctions after age 40: the global study of sexual attitudes and behaviours. Urology 2004 64: 991-997.

# Section 5

# Lifestyle and erectile function

# SMOKING AND IMPOTENCE

## CLINICAL BOTTOM LINE

There is clear linkage between higher rates of smoking and increased erectile dysfunction. Heavy smoking in young men is ten times more common in those with erectile dysfunction before age 45 years than in the general population.

---

One of the real problems with giving advice about smoking to young men is that we are telling them not to smoke now because of health problems they may experience decades in the future. Perhaps a more direct approach on cigarette packets would be more helpful. Not 'smoking kills' but rather 'smoking makes you impotent, then kills you'. A new systematic review of smoking prevalence among impotent men points in that direction [1].

## SYSTEMATIC REVIEW

The review searched MEDLINE from 1980 to about 2000 for articles on impotence or erectile dysfunction and which described studies in the United States. Limiting studies to the US allowed for correlation with available smoking prevalence data for the general population. From each study the number of impotent men who were current smokers, the definition of impotence, the definition of smoking, ages, and location were taken.

For each study, a tailored comparison group based on age distribution, time and location was derived from smoking prevalence data from an ongoing surveillance system.

## RESULTS

There were 19 studies with 3,819 impotent men, ranging in size from 10 to 800 men. Studies usually had a wide age range, with mean age from 35 to 61 years.

In 16 of the 19 studies, smoking rates in impotent men were higher than those in the general male population (Figure 5.1). Overall the age and location matched smoking prevalence in men was 28%. In impotent men it was 40%, a significant difference of 12% (95% confidence interval 11 to 14%).

**FIGURE 5.1: L'ABBÉ PLOT OF SMOKING RATES IN IMPOTENT MEN AND GENERAL MALE POPULATION**

Impotent men who smoke (%)

Smoking men in general population (%)

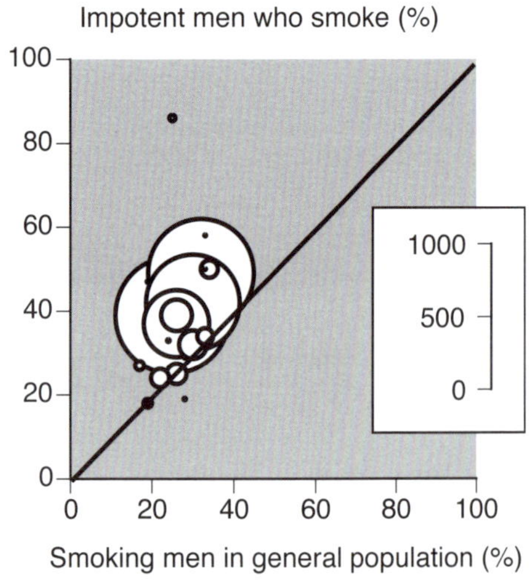

The difference between smoking rates in impotent men and the general male population of 12% was accurately measured by the larger, but not the smaller studies (Figure 5.2). With over 400 men in a study the difference was consistent. With fewer than 100 men the difference ranged from 60% to -9%.

## COMMENT

This paper alone does not constitute a definitive link between smoking and impotence in men. But it does go a long way to making the claim, and in the end it may be more influential in terms of making young men think twice about starting smoking, and make older men think about giving it up. Women may also appreciate the information.

### SMOKING AND ERECTILE DYSFUNCTION

There are at least two systematic reviews of smoking and erectile dysfunction published in 2001 [2, 3]. The bottom line from these is that smoking doubles the risk of erectile dysfunction in men. Erectile problems are common in men, affecting 10-25%. All the evidence may not yet be in, but men might like to work on the basis that smoking will exacerbate a problem that age and chronic disease will bring to their door at some time.

FIGURE 5.2: DIFFERENCE IN SMOKING PREVALENCE IN IMPOTENT MEN AND GENERAL MALE POPULATION BY STUDY SIZE (VERTICAL LINE REPRESENTS OVERALL EXCESS PREVALENCE OF IMPOTENCE IN SMOKERS)

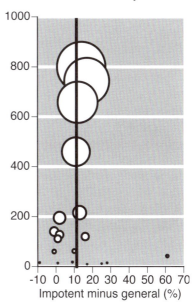

Number of men in study

Impotent minus general (%)

The evidence that smoking history is strongly related to erectile dysfunction continues to build in studies from Finland [4] and Italy [5]. Recovery from erectile dysfunction may be more difficult in smokers or ex-smokers, and duration of smoking habit increases the risk of erectile dysfunction. A further Italian study [6] showed that smoking more than 20 cigarettes a day was very much more common in men aged 18-44 years with erectile dysfunction (39%) than in the Italian population as a whole, where it was 4% for men of the same age.

### REFERENCES:

1. TO Tengs, ND Osgood. The link between smoking and impotence: two decades of evidence. Preventative Medicine 2001 32: 447-452.

2.  KT McVary et al. Smoking and erectile dysfunction: evidence based analysis. Journal of Urology 2001 166:1624-1632.
3.  G Dorey. Is smoking a cause of erectile dysfunction? A literature review. British Journal of Nursing 2001 10:455-65.
4.  R Shiri et al. Relationship between smoking and erectile dysfunction. International Journal of Impotence Research 2005 17: 164-169.
5.  V Mirone et al. Cigarette smoking as risk factor for erectile dysfunction: results from an Italian epidemiological study. European Urology 2002 41: 294-297.
6.  A Natali et al. Heavy smoking is an important risk factor for erectile dysfunction in young men. International Journal of Impotence Research 2005 17: 227-230.

# Erectile dysfunction and lifestyle

## Clinical bottom line

The only modifiable risk factor for erectile dysfunction is having a BMI over 30.

---

Erectile dysfunction is common, affecting a significant proportion of older men, and it increases with older age. There is little known about lifestyle factors and erectile dysfunction, although losing weight helps about a quarter of younger men with a mean weight of 100 kg or more.

## Study

The population for this study [1] was 3,152 men born in 1924, 1934, or 1944 living in Tampere, Finland, in 1994. They were asked a series of questions in 1994, and five years later, by means of a mailed questionnaire, which had questions about erectile function.

Erectile dysfunction had predetermined criteria, basically the inability to achieve or maintain an erection sufficient for satisfactory sexual function. Incidence was calculated by dividing the number of new cases between surveys by the number of person years of follow up.

**FIGURE 5.3: ANNUAL INCIDENCE OF ERECTILE DYSFUNCTION ACCORDING TO AGE**

Annual incidence per 1000 person years

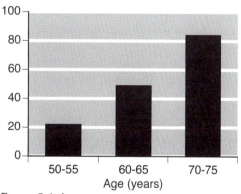

## Results

There were 1130 men free of erectile dysfunction in 1994, half 50 years old, 37% 60 years old, and 13% 70 years old. Most were married or living with a partner. A fifth were current smokers, and 17% had a body mass index of 30 or more.

The incidence of erectile dysfunction increased with age, and doubled for each decade (Figure 5.3). Erectile dysfunction was not related to marital status, smok-

**FIGURE 5.4: ANNUAL INCIDENCE OF ERECTILE DYSFUNCTION ACCORDING TO BMI**

Annual incidence per 1000 person years

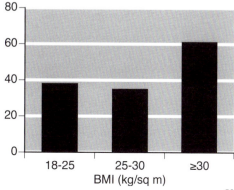

ing alcohol, or coffee intake, but was related to being overweight with a BMI of above 30 (Figure 5.4).

## COMMENT

Age is something we can do nothing about. Not getting overweight is controllable, and this observational study is in accord with a randomised trial showing that losing weight improves erectile function.

It is quite interesting that there are relatively few studies about erectile dysfunction and lifestyle, and those sometimes come to different conclusions, as with smoking in this and the previous study. While there are obvious medical risk factors, like prostate or lower abdominal surgery or trauma, some others, like diabetes or arterial disease, themselves have risk factors, many of which are modifiable (smoking and being overweight high among them).

Healthy living comes down to simple rules, like not smoking, not being overweight, being active, and eating and drinking sensibly, especially fresh fruit and vegetables, and regular but moderate alcohol. The evidence we have is that healthy living not only stops you having heart disease, cancer, and a whole host of other problems, but that if you are a young or younger man, it also protects and maintains your sexual potency.

### REFERENCE

1. R Shiri et al. Effect of life-style factors on incidence of erectile dysfunction. International Journal of Impotence Research 2004 16: 389-394.

# Weight loss and erectile function

## Clinical bottom line

In younger overweight men with erectile dysfunction, losing weight is highly effective at restoring erectile function.

Is fat sexy? Perhaps it depends on one's perspective, but we have seen that in overweight men there are high reported levels of erectile dysfunction, and that risk of erectile dysfunction increases with increasing BMI. The implication is that losing weight would restore or improve erectile function, and a randomised trial [1] shows that to be the case.

## Randomised trial [1]

This Italian study enrolled young men between 35 and 55 years from a weight loss clinic in Naples. For inclusion they had to have an International Index of Erectile Function (IIEF) score of 21 points or less out of the maximum of 25. The IIEF (p 27) has five questions on erectile function, each scored on a scale of 1 to 5. Scores of 21 or below are indicative of erectile dysfunction. Use of drugs for erectile function was an exclusion criterion.

Men were randomly assigned to a control group or to detailed advice about how to achieve a body weight reduction of 10% or more, with instruction about caloric intake, setting goals, and self-monitoring, with monthly small group sessions. Behavioural and psychological counselling was also available. The goal was a diet containing 1700 kcal daily for the first year, and 1900 daily for the second, and with targets for carbohydrates, protein, unsaturated fats, and fibre.

Men in the control group were given general oral and written information about healthy food choice and exercise at every visit, but without specific individualised programmes. Detailed measurements were made at various times over two years, to include blood tests, food diaries, and erectile function.

## Results

The intervention and control groups (55 men in each) were similar at baseline, with an average age of 43 years, weight of 102 kg, and BMI of 36. At two years the control group had virtually no change in caloric intake, while men in the intervention group had an average of 340 kcal less every day, and also took much more daily exercise. Men in the intervention group increased their intake of fibre, protein, and unsaturated fat, and decreased their consumption of saturated fat and cholesterol.

The result was that in the intervention group men lost an average of 15 kg, their BMI fell to 31, and they developed a waist. In the control group there was no change in average weight or in IIEF score, while in the intervention group weight loss and improvement in IIEF score were proportionate (Figure 5.5).

By the end of two years, three of 55 men (5%) in the control group who originally had IIEF scores of 21 or less now had scores of 22 or greater. In the intervention group, 17 men (31%) now had scores of 22 or greater, indicating that they did not have erectile dysfunction. The number needed to treat for weight loss to restore erectile function was 3.9 (95% CI 2.6 to 8.4)

There were significant improvements in blood pressure (by about 3 mmHg on average), total and high density cholesterol, triglycerides, fasting glucose, C-reactive protein and other variables in men in the intervention group with weight loss.

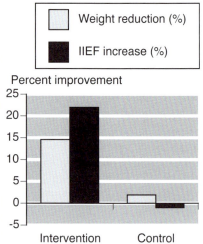

FIGURE 5.5: CHANGE IN AVERAGE WEIGHT AND IIEF SCORES OVER TWO YEARS IN MEN ON INTENSIVE WEIGHT LOSS PROGRAMME OR CONTROL

## COMMENT

Observational studies linking overweight to erectile dysfunction in men create a hypothesis that losing weight could restore erectile function. The randomised trial may be small in numbers, but was impeccable in detail, and had a very positive result. The NNT of 4 was an intention-to-treat value based on all men randomised, despite about six withdrawing, three in each group. The intensive behavioural intervention produced big weight reductions, and a significant minority of men had restored erectile function. Their average weight was still 88 kg after two years, and BMI was 31 after two years, so even more men may have benefited with continuing weight loss.

Thinner meant more sex, or opportunity for it, in these young men, as well as overall better health. These are important lessons about how overweight is bad, and proper weight is good. A clear message is developing that for those people who are overweight, structured weight loss can restore better health.

### REFERENCE:

1    K Eposito et al. Effect of lifestyle changes on erectile dysfunction in obese men. A randomized controlled trial. JAMA 2004 291: 2978-2984.

# Serum cholesterol and erectile dysfunction

## Clinical bottom line

Hyperlipidaemia appears to be somewhat more common in men with erectile dysfunction. Lowering cholesterol is a good thing in itself, and may improve erectile function in some men. The main message is that keeping cholesterol low may well be good for erectile function as well as for other reasons.

---

## Background

Being overweight is known to be associated with erectile dysfunction. Being overweight is also associated with raised serum cholesterol levels.

## Search

A brief search looked in PubMed for studies of any design published between 2001 and 2005.

## Results

Four studies appeared to be relevant, and are summarised in Table 5.1. Two of them showed elevated total or LDL cholesterol, or both, in men with erectile dysfunction compared with men without erectile dysfunction of similar age. Another had high rates of higher LDL cholesterol.

A fourth study examined the effects of lowering cholesterol levels with statin in a very small number of men with raised cholesterol as their only risk factor for erectile dysfunction. Most had improved erections, and penile function tests also improved.

## Comment

This is not surprising, and there is even speculation that erectile dysfunction could be an early sign of vascular disease in men, as it is associated with being overweight and sedentary, unless there is a specific cause for ED (like prostate surgery). However, this limited amount of evidence has to be contrasted with suggestions of increased reporting of erectile dysfunction in men on cholesterol-lowering drugs, though again without much evidence. This is confusing, and it needs more focused studies to elucidate what is going on.

TABLE 5.1: STUDIES OF SERUM CHOLESTEROL AND ERECTILE DYSFUNCTION (ED)

| Reference | Study | Main results |
|---|---|---|
| M Nikoobakht et al. Int J Impot Res 2005 17: 523-526 Iran | Comparison of lipid profile of 100 men with organic ED with 100 healthy individuals, mean age 44 years. | Significantly higher total and LDL cholesterol in ED group, but not HDL or triglyceride Odds ratio for total cholesterol >6.2 mmol/L was 1.7, and HDL >4.1 mmo/L was 2.0 |
| EA Saltzman et al. J Urol 2004 172: 255-258 USA | 18 men had raised cholesterol as their only risk factor for ED, and 9 participated in the study. Their mean age was 50 years. Atorvastatin for about 4 months decreased serum cholesterol | 8 of 9 had improved erections, and IIEF Erectile function scores rose from average of 14 to 21. There was increased penile rigidity. |
| T Roumeguere et al. Eur Urol 2003 44: 355-359. Belgium | 215 men with ED were compared with 100 men without ED, mean age 60 years | Prevalence of total cholesterol >5.2 mmol/L was 71% in ED vs 52% in normal men Increased CHD risk 57% of ED men, 33% in normal men |
| MK Walczak et al. J Gend Speciif Med 2002 5: 19-24 USA | 154 men with ED recruited, and underwent full examination | 74% had LDL cholesterol above 3.1 mmol/L, and 79% had BMI above 26 |

# Cholesterol-lowering Drugs and Erectile Dysfunction

## Clinical bottom line

Both fibrates and statins appear to be associated with erectile dysfunction, though very infrequently. Switching drugs may be beneficial if erectile dysfunction occurs.

## Review [1]

The review process involved searching eight electronic databases for any reports linking erectile dysfunction or impotence in men with the use of cholesterol lowering drugs. National regulatory adverse drug reaction registers were also examined.

### Results

- Case reports linked both fibrates and statins with erectile dysfunction in a small number of men.
- Review articles linked fibrates with erectile dysfunction.
- Data from randomised clinical trials showed no difference between simvastatin and placebo in the 4S study (37/1814 on simvastatin, 28 of 1803 on placebo), but erectile dysfunction was not reported in other randomised trials.
- One case-control study looked at the prevalence of erectile dysfunction in 339 patients attending a lipid clinic compared with with matched controls. Both fibrates and statins were independent predictors of erectile dysfunction with odds ratios of about 1.5 [2].
- Regulatory agencies in Australia and the UK had yellow card reports of erectile dysfunction in men on lipid lowering drugs, both fibrates and statins. In a small number of men, withdrawal of the lipid-lowering drug and rechallenge resulted in recurrent symptoms, though the rechallenge was usually not blind.

### Comment

This is an interesting paper because it attempts to systematically review adverse events, a subject too often ignored. It identified a number of cases, but in total these were small compared to the very widespread prescribing of lipid lowering drugs, especially statins. It is made more complicated by the average age of men reporting erectile dysfunction, mainly in their 50s when erectile dysfunction may occur anyway, and because many men using statins may be on therapy for other conditions.

One useful observation was that drug switching resolved the problem in a number of cases.

**REFERENCES:**

1   K Rizvi et al. Do lipid-lowering drugs cause erectile dysfunction? A systematic review. Family Practice 2002 19: 95-98.

2   E Bruckert et al. Men treated with hypolipidaemic drugs complain more frequently of erectile dysfunction. Journal of Clinical Pharmacology and Therapy 1996 21: 89-94.

# Herbal erectile dysfunction treatments adulterated

## Clinical bottom line

Two of seven herbal products for erectile dysfunction contained significant doses of PDE-5 inhibitors, equivalent to 30 mg sildenafil and 20 mg tadalafil. This is potentially dangerous for some men with contraindications for PDE-5 inhibitor use.

---

Many people turn to herbal therapies because they are "natural". So they may be, but there is no evidence that any herbal therapy substantially benefits erectile function.

## Study

This study [1] obtained samples of seven different types of herbal treatments for erectile dysfunction, six from the internet. All were oral tablets or capsules, and claimed efficacy if taken before sexual activity. The tablets were crushed, extracted, and examined using high performance liquid chromatography with mass spectrometry. Samples of sildenafil, tadalafil, and vardenafil were also tested.

## Results

One of the seven samples (called super-X) was adulterated with sildenafil, and the average amount of sildenafil per capsule was 30 mg.

Another of the seven samples (called Stamina-Rx) was adulterated with tadalafil, and the average amount of tadalafil per tablet was 20 mg.

## Comment

These are effective doses of PDE-5 inhibitors, and that is probably why some herbal therapies work. This is dangerous, because some men, particularly those on nitrates, have potentially serious reactions with PDE-5 inhibitors. An accompanying editorial comment calls this a "compelling condemnation of the absence of regulation of the nutraceutical industry". It is not an isolated case; several forms of herbal therapy are known to have been adulterated with potent medicines.

### Reference

1    N Fleshner et al. Evidence for contamination of herbal erectile dysfunction products with phosphodiesterase type 5 inhibitors. Journal of Urology 2005 174: 636-641.

# BANDOLIER'S 10 TIPS FOR HEALTHY LIVING

These 10 tips for healthy living have been developed from good evidence, usually meta-analyses of larger observational studies. Many of these tips can help to avoid more than one medical condition. Keeping well has enormously more impact than anything doctors can do for us. Treatment for cancer, heart disease, or hypertension, we have it, and the treatments are not always effective, and frequently unpleasant. Keep away from illness. These ten tips apply just as much for erectile function as heart disease or cancer. Those who follow them probably won't need to read the next couple of sections.

1   Eat whole grain foods (bread, or rice, or pasta) on four occasions a week. This will reduce the chance of having almost any cancer by 40%. Given that cancer gets about 1 in 3 of us in a lifetime, that's big advice.

2   Don't smoke. If you do smoke, stop. If you can't stop, try to reduce your smoking, as there is a profound dose-response (the more you smoke, the more likely you are to have cancer, or heart or respiratory disease), so cut down to below five cigarettes a day and leave long portions of the day without a cigarette.

3   Eat at least five portions of vegetables and fruit a day, and especially tomatoes (including ketchup), red grapes and the like, and salad all year. This protects against a whole variety of different nasty things:
    • It reduces the risk of stroke dramatically
    • It reduces the risk of diabetes considerably
    • It will reduce the risk of heart disease and cancer.

4   Use Benecol or its equivalent instead of butter or margarine. It really does reduce cholesterol, and reducing cholesterol will reduce the risk of heart attack and stroke even in those whose cholesterol is not particularly high.

5   Drink alcohol regularly. The type of alcohol probably doesn't matter too much, but the equivalent of a couple of glasses of wine a day or a couple of beers is a good thing. The odd day without alcohol won't hurt either. Think of it as medicine.

6   Eat fish. Eating fish once a week won't stop you having a heart attack in itself, but it reduces the likelihood of you dying from it by half.

7   Take a multivitamin tablet every day, but be sure that it is one with at least 200 micrograms of folate. The evidence is that this can substantially reduce chances of heart disease in some individuals, and it has been shown to reduce colon cancer by

over 85%. It may also reduce the likelihood of developing dementia. Folate is essential in any woman contemplating pregnancy because it will reduce the chance of some birth defects.

8   If you are pregnant or have high blood pressure, coffee is best minimised. For the rest of us drinking four cups of coffee a day is likely to reduce our chances of getting colon cancer and Parkinson's disease.

9   Get breathless more often. You don't have to go to a gym or be an Olympic marathon runner. Simply walking a mile a day, or taking reasonable exercise three times a week (enough to make you sweat or glow) will substantially reduce the risk of heart disease. If you walk, don't dawdle. Make it a brisk pace. One of the benefits of regular exercise is that it strengthens bones and keeps them strong. Breaking a hip when elderly is a very serious thing.

10  Check your height and weight on a chart to see if you are overweight for your height. Your body mass index is the weight in kilograms divided by the height in metres squared: for preference it should be below 25. If you are overweight, lose it. This has many benefits. There is no good evidence on simple ways to lose weight that work. Crash diets don't work. Take it one step at a time, do the things that are possible now, and combine some calorie limitation with increased exercise.

# SECTION 6

# PDE-5 INHIBITORS FOR ERECTILE DYSFUNCTION

## Clinical Bottom Line

Sildenafil has been studied in a large number of men, with many different causes of their erectile dysfunction, and in different parts of the world. At the top fixed doses of 50 or 100 mg, or in the dose-optimised schedule of 25-100 mg, it has considerable efficacy, with a number needed to treat below 2, and 76% of men have improved erections. Headache (17%), flushing (13%), dyspepsia (8%), and rhinitis (5%) were the most common individual adverse events, though few men discontinued because of adverse events.

---

## Reference

RA Moore et al. Indirect comparison of interventions using published randomised trials: Systematic review of PDE-5 inhibitors for erectile dysfunction. BMC Urology 2005 5:18.

## Systematic Review

Randomised trials were sought of three PDE-5 inhibitors (sildenafil, tadalafil, vardenafil), with placebo or active comparator, in men with erectile dysfunction of any causation, with drugs used at home. Previous systematic reviews were used to source trials or trial data, supplemented by electronic searches of PubMed (to June 2005, and supplemented by searches to November 2005 for this update) and the Cochrane Library (issue 1, 2005) using drug names and randomis(z)ed trial.

Information extracted was efficacy, using a number of different efficacy outcomes, discontinuations, and specific adverse events. Because various dosing regimens were used, including fixed doses, and dose-optimised regimens, and because there was a similarity of result for the top two fixed doses (50 and 100 mg) and dose optimised (25-100 mg), where most men used 50 or 100 mg), results here include all studies reporting on 50 mg, 100 mg, or dose optimised regimens.

- Date review completed: June 2005, updated November 2005

- Number of trials included: Maximum efficacy data on 30 trials, but 37 in all

- Number of patients: 5,599 men in largest analysis, but 7,500 men in total

- Control groups: Placebo

- Main outcomes: Improved erections, IIEF, discontinuations, specific adverse events

## RESULTS

None of the trials used an active comparator, and most scored highly on reporting quality – all were randomised and double blind for inclusion in the review. Most studies were in men with erectile dysfunction of mixed aetiology, but trials were also conducted in men with diabetes, depression, spinal cord injury, coronary heart disease, radiotherapy for prostate cancer, renal failure and haemodialysis, rectal surgery, and spina bifida. Studies were conducted worldwide, including Europe, North and South America, Asia, and Africa.

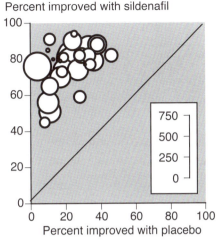

FIGURE 6.1: IMPROVED ERECTIONS IN COMPARISONS OF SILDENAFIL AND PLACEBO

ERECTILE FUNCTION

With sildenafil 50/100 mg, the erectile function domain score rose to 22 (compared with 14 for placebo), an average 10-point change. Successful attempts at intercourse occurred 65% of the time, compared with 23% with placebo.

On average, in 5,599 men in 30 trials, 76% of men reported improved erections, compared with 23% with placebo (Figure 6.1). The number needed to treat for one man to have improved erections compared with placebo was 1.9 (95% confidence interval 1.8 to 2.0; Table 6.1 overpage).

ADVERSE EVENTS

All-cause discontinuation and lack of efficacy discontinuation were less frequent with sildenafil than placebo, but adverse event discontinuation more frequent. About 1% more men discontinued because of adverse events with sildenafil than with placebo (Table 6.1 overpage).

About half of men had some adverse event, but serious adverse events were no more common with sildenafil than with placebo in these trials. Headache (17%), flushing (13%), dyspepsia (8%), and rhinitis (5%) were the most common individual adverse events.

## COMMENT

Sildenafil has been studied in a large number of men, with many different causes of their erectile dysfunction, and in different parts of the world. At the top fixed doses of 50 or

| Outcome | Number of | | Percent with | | Relative benefit or risk (95% CI) | NNT/NNTp/NNH (95% CI) |
|---|---|---|---|---|---|---|
| | Trials | Patients | Sildenafil | Placebo | | |
| **Efficacy** | | | | | | |
| Improved erections | 30 | 5599 | 76 | 23 | 3.3 (3.1 to 3.6) | 1.9 (1.8 to 2.0) |
| **Discontinuation** | | | | | | |
| All-cause | 29 | 5343 | 8.2 | 12 | 0.7 (0.6 to 0.8) | **28 (19 to 50)** |
| Lack of efficacy | 29 | 5228 | 1.2 | 4.4 | 0.3 (0.2 to 0.5) | **32 (25 to 45)** |
| Adverse event | 30 | 5554 | 1.6 | 0.6 | 1.8 (1.2 to 2.7) | **110 (64 to 450)** |
| **Adverse events** | | | | | | |
| All cause | 17 | 2634 | 49 | 29 | 1.7 (1.5 to 1.8) | **4.9 (4.2 to 6.0)** |
| Serious | 16 | 2364 | 1.6 | 1.6 | 1.0 (0.6 to 1.7) | not calculated |
| Headache | 33 | 6166 | 17 | 5.2 | 3.3 (2.8 to 3.9) | **8.8 (7.7 to 10)** |
| Dyspepsia | 25 | 4740 | 7.9 | 2.4 | 3.2 (2.4 to 4.3) | **18 (15 to 24)** |
| Flushing | 32 | 6135 | 13 | 1.7 | 6.6 (5.1 to 8.5) | **9.1 (8.2 to 10)** |
| Rhinitis | 20 | 4057 | 5.4 | 1.8 | 2.4 (1.7 to 3.4) | **32 (23 to 50)** |

NNT is given in standard font, **NNTp in bold**, and **NNH in bold in shaded boxes**.
No NNT/NNTp/NNH was calculated unless there was a statistically significant difference

100 mg, or in the dose-optimised schedule of 25-100 mg, it has considerable efficacy, with a number needed to treat below 2. To have such good efficacy despite the wide range of conditions studied indicates a robust result.

OTHER SYSTEMATIC REVIEWS OF SILDENAFIL

1. RA Moore et al. Sildenafil (Viagra) for male erectile dysfunction: a meta-analysis of clinical trial reports. BMC Urology 2002 2:6. (www.biomedcentral.com/1471-2490/2/6/).
2. A Burls et al. Systematic review of randomized controlled trials of sildenafil (Viagra®) in the treatment of male erectile dysfunction. British Journal of General Practice 2001 51: 1004-1012.
3. HA Fink et al. Sildenafil for male erectile dysfunction: a systematic review and meta-analysis. Archives of Internal Medicine 2002 162:1349-1360.

# Tadalafil for erectile dysfunction – 2005 update

## Clinical bottom line

Tadalafil has been studied in a large number of men. At the fixed doses of 10 or 20 mg, it has considerable efficacy, with a number needed to treat below 2, and 75% of men have improved erections. Headache (13%), dyspepsia (10%), flushing (5%), and rhinitis (3%) were the most common individual adverse events.

---

### Reference

RA Moore et al. Indirect comparison of interventions using published randomised trials: Systematic review of PDE-5 inhibitors for erectile dysfunction. BMC Urology 2005 5:18.

### Systematic review

Randomised trials were sought of three PDE-5 inhibitors (sildenafil, tadalafil, vardenafil), with placebo or active comparator, in men with erectile dysfunction of any causation, with drugs used at home. Previous systematic reviews were used to source trials or trial data, supplemented by electronic searches of PubMed (to June 2005, and supplemented by searches to November 2005 for this update) and the Cochrane Library (issue 1, 2005) using drug names and randomis(z)ed trial.

Information extracted was efficacy, using a number of different efficacy outcomes, discontinuations, and specific adverse events. Almost all information was for the 20 mg dose, with a small amount for the 10 mg dose; information was combined for 10 and 20 mg.

- Date review completed: June 2005, updated November 2005

- Number of trials included: Maximum data on 8 trials, but 10 in all

- Number of patients: 1,694 men in largest analysis, but 2,330 men in total

- Control groups: Placebo

- Main outcomes: Improved erections, IIEF, discontinuations, specific adverse events

RESULTS

None of the trials used an active comparator, and most scored highly on reporting quality – all were randomised and double blind for inclusion in the review. Most of the studies used an enriched enrolment in which previous unsuccessful treatment with a PDE-5 inhibitor was an exclusion criterion.

Most studies were in men with erectile dysfunction of mixed aetiology, diabetes, or following prostatectomy. Studies were conducted mainly in Europe and North America.

ERECTILE FUNCTION

With tadalafil 10/20 mg, the erectile function domain score rose to 22 (compared with 15 for placebo), an average 8-point change. Successful attempts at intercourse occurred 62% of the time, compared with 26% with placebo.

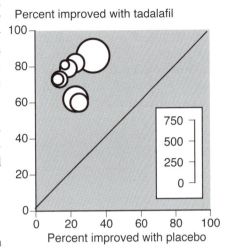

On average, in 1,694 men in 8 trials, 75% of men reported improved erections, compared with 23% with placebo (Figure 6.2). The number needed to treat for one man to have improved erections compared with placebo was 1.9 (95% confidence interval 1.8 to 2.1; Table 6.2).

ADVERSE EVENTS

All-cause discontinuation and lack of efficacy discontinuation were less frequent with tadalafil than placebo, but adverse event discontinuation more frequent. About 2% more men discontinued because of adverse events with tadalafil than with placebo (Table 6.2).

About half of men had some adverse event, but serious adverse events were no more common with tadalafil than with placebo in these trials. Headache (13%), dyspepsia (10%), flushing (5%), and rhinitis (3%) were the most common individual adverse events.

COMMENT

Tadalafil has been studied in a large number of men. At the fixed doses of 10 or 20 mg, it has considerable efficacy, with a number needed to treat below 2.

TABLE 6.2: EFFICACY AND ADVERSE EVENT OUTCOMES IN TRIALS OF TADALAFIL AND PLACEBO

| Outcome | Number of | | Percent with | | Relative benefit or risk (95% CI) | NNT/NNTp/NNH (95% CI) |
|---|---|---|---|---|---|---|
| | Trials | Patients | Tadalafil | Placebo | | |
| **Efficacy** | | | | | | |
| Improved erections | 8 | 1694 | 75 | 23 | 3.2 (2.8 to 3.8) | 1.9 (1.8 to 2.1) |
| **Discontinuation** | | | | | | |
| All-cause | 5 | 1334 | 13 | 19 | 0.7 (0.5 to 0.9) | 15 (8.8 to 46) |
| Lack of efficacy | 6 | 1432 | 3.3 | 7.5 | 0.5 (0.3 to 0.7) | 24 (14 to 69) |
| Adverse event | 7 | 1655 | 3.4 | 1.5 | 2.3 (1.1 to 5.1) | 52 (29 to 260) |
| **Adverse events** | | | | | | |
| All cause | 3 | 590 | 47 | 25 | 1.8 (1.4 to 2.3) | 4.6 (3.4 to 7.2) |
| Serious | 7 | 1651 | 1.2 | 1.1 | 1.0 (0.4 to 2.8) | not calculated |
| Headache | 7 | 1810 | 13 | 3.4 | 3.5 (2.2 to 5.4) | 11 (8.5 to 14) |
| Dyspepsia | 6 | 1396 | 10 | 0.2 | 12 (4.3 to 35) | 11 (8.8 to 14) |
| Flushing | 6 | 1525 | 4.8 | 0.2 | 7.2 (2.5 to 20) | 24 (18 to 38) |
| Rhinitis | 2 | 711 | 3.1 | 0.5 | 4.5 (0.8 to 24) | not calculated |

NNT is given in standard font, **NNTp in bold**, and **NNH in bold in shaded boxes**. No NNT/NNTp/NNH was calculated unless there was a statistically significant difference

OTHER SYSTEMATIC REVIEWS OF TADALAFIL

1. CC Carson et al. The efficacy and safety of tadalafil: an update. BJU International 2004 93: 1276-1281.

## Clinical bottom line

Vardenafil has been studied in a large number of men. At the fixed doses of 10 or 20 mg or in a dose optimised regimen, it has considerable efficacy, with a number needed to treat of about 2. Headache (15%), flushing (13%), rhinitis (8%), and dyspepsia (4%), were the most common individual adverse events.

---

### Reference

RA Moore et al. Indirect comparison of interventions using published randomised trials: Systematic review of PDE-5 inhibitors for erectile dysfunction. BMC Urology 2005 5:18.

### Systematic review

Randomised trials were sought of three PDE-5 inhibitors (sildenafil, tadalafil, vardenafil), with placebo or active comparator, in men with erectile dysfunction of any causation, with drugs used at home. Previous systematic reviews were used to source trials or trial data, supplemented by electronic searches of PubMed (to June 2005, and supplemented by searches to November 2005 for this update) and the Cochrane Library (issue 1, 2005) using drug names and randomis(z)ed trial.

Information extracted was efficacy, using a number of different efficacy outcomes, discontinuations, and specific adverse events. Almost all information was for the 10 and 20 mg dose, and a dose optimised regimen; information was combined for 10 and 20 mg fixed dose, and for the dose optimised regimen.

- Date review completed: June 2005, updated November 2005

- Number of trials included: Maximum data on 8 trials, but 9 in all

- Number of patients: 3,379 men in largest analysis, but 4,324 men in total

- Control groups: Placebo

- Main outcomes: Improved erections, IIEF, discontinuations, specific adverse events

None of the trials used an active comparator, and most scored highly on reporting quality – all were randomised and double blind for inclusion in the review. Most of the studies used an enriched enrolment in which previous unsuccessful treatment with a PDE-5 inhibitor was an exclusion criterion.

Most studies were in men with erectile dysfunction of mixed aetiology, diabetes, or following prostatectomy. Studies were conducted mainly in Europe and North America.

### ERECTILE FUNCTION

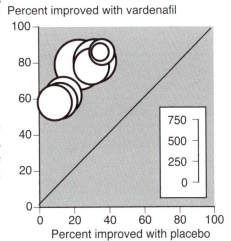

FIGURE **6.3:** IMPROVED ERECTIONS IN COMPARISONS OF VARDENAFIL AND PLACEBO

With vardenafil 10/20 mg, the erectile function domain score rose to 20 (compared with 14 for placebo), an average 8-point change. Successful attempts at intercourse occurred 59% of the time, compared with 28% with placebo.

On average, in 3,379 men in 8 trials, 72% of men reported improved erections, compared with 24% with placebo (Figure 6.3). The number needed to treat for one man to have improved erections compared with placebo was 2.1 (95% confidence interval 1.9 to 2.2; Table 6.3, overpage).

### ADVERSE EVENTS

All-cause discontinuation and lack of efficacy discontinuation were less frequent with vardenafil than placebo, but adverse event discontinuation more frequent. About 1% more men discontinued because of adverse events with vardenafil than with placebo (Table 6.3, overpage).

The proportion of men with at least one adverse event was not reported in these trials, but serious adverse events were no more common with vardenafil than with placebo. Headache (15%), flushing (13%), rhinitis (8%), and dyspepsia (4%), were the most common individual adverse events.

| Outcome | Number of | | Percent with | | Relative benefit or risk (95% CI) | NNT/NNTp/NNH (95%CI) |
|---|---|---|---|---|---|---|
| | Trials | Patients | Vardenafil | Placebo | | |
| **Efficacy** | | | | | | |
| Improved erections | 8 | 3379 | 72 | 24 | 3.1 (2.8 to 3.5) | 2.1 (1.9 to 2.2) |
| **Withdrawal** | | | | | | |
| All-cause | 5 | 2061 | 20 | 32 | 0.6 (0.5 to 0.6) | **7.7 (6.0 to 11)** |
| Lack of efficacy | 6 | 2320 | 4 | 12 | 0.3 (0.2 to 0.4) | **11 (9.0 to 16)** |
| Adverse event | 7 | 2868 | 3.3 | 1.8 | 1.8 (1.1 to 3.0) | **65 (37 to 250)** |
| **Adverse events** | | | | | | |
| All cause | | | insufficient data | | | |
| Severe | 3 | 1095 | 2.7 | 2.2 | 1.2 (0.5 to 2.8) | not calculated |
| Serious | 5 | 1983 | 2.2 | 3.2 | 0.7 ( 0.4 to 1.2) | not calculated |
| Headache | 6 | 2411 | 15 | 4.1 | 3.4 (2.4 to 4.8) | **9.6 (7.9 to 12)** |
| Dyspepsia | 5 | 1969 | 3.8 | 0.3 | 7.3 (2.4 to 22) | **31 (22 to 48)** |
| Flushing | 5 | 1982 | 13 | 0.8 | 13 (6.3 to 27) | **8.0 (6.9 to 9.6)** |
| Rhinitis | 5 | 2211 | 7.9 | 3.6 | 2.2 (1.5 to 3.4) | **23 (16 to 42)** |

NNT is given in standard font, **NNTp in bold**, and **NNH in bold in shaded boxes**.
No NNT/NNTp/NNH was calculated unless there was a statistically significant difference

COMMENT

Vardenafil has been studied in a large number of men. At the fixed doses of 10 or 20 mg or in a dose optimised regimen, it has considerable efficacy, with a number needed to treat of about 2.

OTHER SYSTEMATIC REVIEWS OF VARDENAFIL

1. S Markou et al. Vardenafil (Levitra) for erectile dysfunction: a systematic review and meta-analysis of clinical trial reports. International Journal of Impotence Research 2004 July doi:10.1038/sj.ijir.3901258 (online publications).

## CLINICAL BOTTOM LINE

Despite enriched enrolment in tadalafil and vardenafil trials, and the greater clinical and geographical variation for sildenafil than tadalafil and vardenafil, results for the three PDE-5 inhibitors were generally similar for efficacy and particular adverse events. Discontinuation rates were somewhat lower for sildenafil.

## SYSTEMATIC REVIEW [1]

Randomised trials were sought of three PDE-5 inhibitors (sildenafil, tadalafil, vardenafil), with placebo or active comparator, in men with erectile dysfunction of any causation, with drugs used at home. Previous systematic reviews were used to source trials or trial data, supplemented by electronic searches of PubMed (to June 2005, and supplemented by searches to November 2005 for this update) and the Cochrane Library (issue 1, 2005) using drug names and randomis(z)ed trial.

Information extracted was of efficacy, using a number of different efficacy outcomes, discontinuations, and specific adverse events. For the comparisons, information is taken for the top two doses used, or any dose optimised regimen that included the top two doses of any PDE-5 inhibitor.

- Date review completed: June 2005

- Number of trials included: 50

- Number of patients: 12,580

- Control groups: placebo

- Main outcomes: Improved erections, IIEF, discontinuations, specific adverse events

## RESULTS

There were more men in sildenafil trials (7,135) than tadalafil (2,071) or vardenafil (3,374). Trials were of generally high reporting quality, and all of them were at a minimum both randomised and double blind. Compared with tadalafil and vardenafil, sildenafil was studied in more clinical conditions, though erectile dysfunction of mixed aetiology or diabetes comprised about 85% of all men in the studies. There was a wider geographical spread with sildenafil, but most studies were in Europe, North America, or Australia. Although various doses were used in the trials, and some dose-optimised regimens for sildenafil and vardenafil, results from the top two doses or dose-optimised regimens were similar for each drug, and pooled.

The analysis therefore aggregates the most information for the three PDE-5 inhibitors. This report shows the results, without any attempt to demonstrate statistical differences between the three PDE-5 inhibitors.

OUTCOMES REPORTED

Table 6.4 shows the outcomes reported, in terms of percentage of men in the trials reporting that outcome. Improved erections and success rates were reported commonly, together with the final score and mean change in the erectile function domain.

Discontinuations, for any reason, or because of adverse events or lack of efficacy, were also commonly reported. Adverse event reporting was less consistent, with some adverse events being reported consistently, and others not. The reason was that adverse events with incidence below 2%-5% were often not reported.

EFFICACY

The erectile function domain score at the end of treatment, and the change in the erectile function domain score for the top doses of all three PDE-5 inhibitors are shown in Figure 6.4. The percentage of men with improved erections, and percentage of successful attempts at intercourse, are shown in Figure 6.5. There is similarity between the three treatments, though with a tendency for slightly better results with sildenafil.

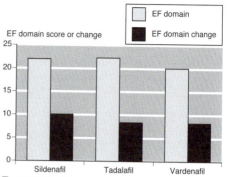

FIGURE 6.4: MEAN ERECTILE FUNCTION SCORES AND MEAN DOMAIN CHANGE

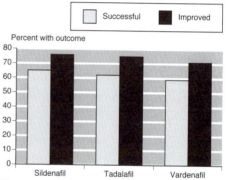

FIGURE 6.5: MEAN PERCENT WITH SUCCESSFUL ATTEMPTS AT INTERCOURSE AND IMPROVED ERECTIONS

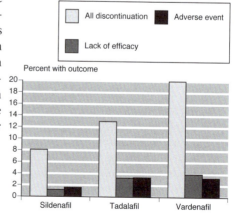

FIGURE 6.6: DISCONTINUATION RATES FOR ANY CAUSE, LACK OF EFFICACY, AND ADVERSE EVENTS

TABLE 6.4: PERCENTAGE OF MEN IN ALL TRIALS FOR WHOM PARTICULAR OUTCOMES WERE SOUGHT, AND WHO FORM THE DENOMINATOR IN REPORTS OF THE TRIALS

| Outcome | Sildenafil n=6860 | Tadalafil n=2036 | Vardenafil n=3274 |
|---|---|---|---|
| **Efficacy** | | | |
| Improved erections | 83 | 83 | 100 |
| Successful attempts at SI | 49 | 72 | 100 |
| Final score IIEF Q3 | 94 | 27 | 26 |
| Mean change IIEF Q3 | 91 | 27 | 26 |
| Final score IIEF Q4 | 94 | 27 | 26 |
| Mean change IIEF Q4 | 91 | 27 | 26 |
| Final score EF Domain | 58 | 72 | 100 |
| Mean change EF Domain | 55 | 83 | 77 |
| **Withdrawals** | | | |
| All-cause | 82 | 65 | 69 |
| Lack of efficacy | 81 | 72 | 82 |
| Adverse event | 89 | 83 | 100 |
| **Adverse events** | | | |
| Men with any adverse event | 40 | 40 | 18 |
| Serious | 36 | 83 | 78 |
| Treatment related | 54 | 3 | 43 |
| Headache | 99 | 90 | 86 |
| Dyspepsia | 78 | 71 | 73 |
| Flushing | 99 | 73 | 73 |
| Nasal congestion/Rhinitis | 62 | 35 | 73 |
| Visual disturbances | 89 | 46 | 55 |
| Cardiovascular events | 25 | 27 | 33 |
| Priapism | 30 | 0 | 0 |

SI - sexual intercourse; EF - erectile function

DISCONTINUATIONS

Figure 6.6 shows discontinuation rates for any cause, for lack of efficacy, and for adverse events for all three PDE-5 inhibitors. Rates were generally lower with sildenafil, though this was also the case with placebo, and the differences may reflect differing expectations over time. Tadalafil and vardenafil were studied in men in whom PDE-5 inhibitors were known to work, and it might have led to less tolerance of adverse events in them.

## PARTICULAR ADVERSE EVENTS

There was no difference in the incidence of serious adverse events between any of the three PDE-5 inhibitors and placebo. Particular adverse events, headache, flushing, dyspepsia and rhinitis were commonly reported, and Figure 6.7 shows the average incidence for each PDE-5 inhibitor. They were generally similar.

FIGURE 6.7: EVENT RATES FOR HEADACHE, FLUSHING, DYSPEPSIA AND RHINITIS

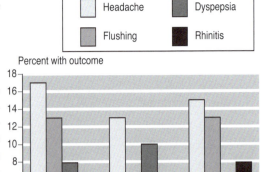

## COMMENT

Perhaps the most obvious difference between trials of different drugs was the use of different exclusion criteria in individual studies. Five of eight tadalafil studies, and six of seven vardenafil studies excluded men previously unresponsive to PDE-5 inhibitors, thus permitting enrolment to be enriched by responders compared with sildenafil studies, in which such an exclusion would not have been used because it was the first available PDE-5 inhibitor. It is not clear how this major difference might have affected the measured performance of the drugs. Exclusion of non-responders to other PDE-5 inhibitors might be expected to enhance the measured performance of any other PDE-5 inhibitor under test, making it look better in indirect comparisons. The NNT would be better under these conditions than it would be for the wider ED population.

Despite this, and despite the greater clinical and geographical variation in sildenafil trials than tadalafil and vardenafil trials, results for the three PDE-5 inhibitors were generally similar for efficacy and particular adverse events. Discontinuation rates were somewhat lower for sildenafil.

REFERENCE:

1    RA Moore et al. Indirect comparison of interventions using published randomised trials: Systematic review of PDE-5 inhibitors for erectile dysfunction. BMC Urology 2005 5:18.

## Clinical bottom line

A large retrospective survey of sildenafil in clinical practice confirms results of clinical trials, with no evidence of rare but serious adverse events.

---

Sildenafil became available in the UK in 1998 for the treatment of erectile dysfunction, a condition most commonly found in older men. At the time there were concerns over possible cardiac effects, and use in men taking nitrates was contraindicated.

## Study [1]

This was a prescription event monitoring study in which exposure data were derived from dispensed prescription details and outcome data from questionnaires returned by GPs. The period was April to August 1999, with questionnaires sent to GPs about 18 months after the date of the first dispensed prescription.

Questionnaires sought information about demographics, dose of sildenafil, reasons for discontinuation if it was stopped, and information about suspected adverse drug reactions. Events would include any new diagnosis, referral to a consultant, or admission to hospital, deterioration or improvement in current illness, alteration in laboratory values, or other complaint of sufficient importance to enter into the patient's notes.

## Results

The number of questionnaires posted was 45,000, and 25,000 (55%) were returned, with useful information on 22,500. The men referred to in these forms had median age of 60 years, with a range of 18 to 92 years. Diabetes was a factor in at least 18% of these men. Sildenafil was reported as effective in 71%.

There were 145 events coded as adverse drug reactions that GPs thought attributable to sildenafil (Table 6.5). These were mainly headache, flushing and dyspepsia. Others included myalgia, priapism, and oedema. There were three cases of palpitations, two of tachycardia, and one each of angina, myocardial infarction, and stroke.

Just under 4000 men stopped taking sildenafil (18%), mostly because of lack of efficacy, though

TABLE 6.5: MAIN ADRs WITH SILDENAFIL

| ADR | Number |
|---|---|
| Headache | 30 |
| Unspecified | 22 |
| Flushing | 16 |
| Dyspepsia | 13 |
| Dizziness | 7 |
| Visual disturbance | 7 |

also because the erectile dysfunction had improved, or because of adverse events or medical conditions.

The leading causes of death were malignancy (122), myocardial infarction (56), and ischaemic heart disease (20). The standardised mortality rate was lower than that for men in England in 1998, but with wide confidence intervals.

## COMMENT

The large and detailed retrospective survey of 22,000 men prescribed sildenafil largely confirms results from the clinical trials. Success was achieved in about 70% or so, with some adverse events, but no evidence of an increased rate of rare, serious adverse events.

### REFERENCE

1   A Boshier et al. Evaluation of the safety of sildenafil for male erectile dysfunction: experience gained in general practice use in England in 1999. BJU International 2004 93:796-801.

# PDE-5 INHIBITORS AFTER PROSTATECTOMY

## CLINICAL BOTTOM LINE

Nerve-sparing surgery results in improved return of sexual function, but over a period of time. Use of PDE-5 inhibitors initially can help.

---

The last two decades have seen much greater focus on prostate cancer. The advent of screening using prostate specific antigen has increased detection rates among younger men. The advent of fitter cohorts of older men, and changes in attitudes, have all meant that there has been increased interest in the maintenance of erectile function after operation.

## REVIEWS

There are two recent reviews [1,2] which chart how surgical techniques have changed, with increasing interest in maintaining the integrity of the cavernous nerves, using the so-called nerve-sparing technique. This discovery offered the possibility of preserving erectile function which was all but totally eliminated before this modification. Experienced surgeons at major academic centres claim recovery rates of satisfactory intercourse of 60-85% in their patients.

Recovery of sexual function is not immediate, however, and it can take up to two years for full recovery even after nerve sparing surgery. Where there is delay, oral PDE-5 inhibitors are usually the first line therapy, with reported efficacy in 10-80% of men after nerve sparing surgery, but probably below 15% after non-nerve sparing surgery. Second line therapies include intraurethral medications, intracavernosal injections and vacuum constriction devices, which should restore erectile function to most men. A systematic review [2] examines the literature on recovery of erectile function after radical prostatectomy, including the prophylactic use of PDE-5 inhibitors to aid recovery of erectile function.

Table 6.6 charts some of the more recent observational studies with sildenafil, and there have been several randomised trials for tadalafil and vardenafil in men following nerve sparing surgery. They all confirm efficacy of PDE-5 inhibitors after this type of surgery.

## REFERENCES

1    AL Burnett. Erectile dysfunction following radical prostatectomy. JAMA 2005 293: 2648-2653.
2    F Montorsi et al. Current and future strategies for preventing and managing erectile dysfunction following radical prostatectomy. European Urology 2004 45: 123-133.

TABLE 6.6: STUDIES OF SILDENAFIL IN MEN AFTER PROSTATECTOMY

| Reference | Patients | Number of men | Outcome |
|---|---|---|---|
| Penson. J Urol 2005 173:1701-1705. | Sample of 1,288 men after radical prostatectomy for cancer. | 554 used sildenafil at some time | At 24 months erections firm enough for intercourse in 22%, and 28% by 60 months. Stable between 2 and 5 years |
| Rubio Briones et al. Actas Urol Esp 2004 28:567-574. | Survey of 111 men after radical prostatectomy taking sildenafil | 90 | Half the men had complete or partial response. Response to sildenafil better after the first year |
| Raina et al. Urology 2003 62:110-115. | Study after radical prostatectomy at 1 and 4 years after surgery on sildenafil 50-100 mg | 91 | 71% of those originally responding were still responding at 3 years. |
| Feng et al. J Urol 2000 164:1935-1938. | Patients after radical prostatectomy taking sildenafil | 53 | 15/21 with bilateral nerve sparing had response, but only 1/17 with non-nerve sparing procedure |
| Blander et al. Int J Impot Res 2000 12:165-168. | Comparison of effects of sildenafil after surgery and without surgery | 107 | Higher success rates without surgery |
| Zagaja et al. Urology 2000 56:631-634. | Men after radical prostatectomy needing sildenafil | 170 | In young men in whom both neurovascular bundles were preserved response rate was 80%. No adequate response in older patients where bundles were removed |
| Zippe et al. Urology 2000 55:241-245. | Men after radical prostatectomy needing sildenafil | 91 | Good response in 72% with bilateral nerve sparing, less with unilateral, and poor without nerve sparing surgery |
| Hong et al Int J Impot Res 1999 11 Supp 1: S15-22. | Men after radical prostatectomy needing sildenafil | 198 | Initial treatment satisfaction rose from 26% at 6 months to 60% at 2 years |
| Lowentritt et al. J Urol 1999 162:1614-1617. | Men after radical prostatectomy needing sildenafil | 84 | Degree of nerve sparing had a significant impact on efficacy of sildenafil |

# PDE-5 INHIBITORS -
## EVIDENCE FROM OTHER STUDIES, RANDOMISED AND NON-RANDOMISED

CLINICAL BOTTOM LINE

There are very considerable amounts of information available in the form of observational studies. For sildenafil, the first drug introduced in this class, there were more than 33,000 men in observational studies, compared with under 4,000 in randomised trials.

---

Evidence from systematic reviews of good quality randomised trials may be the highest form of evidence, but it is not the only evidence available. There are circumstances in which randomisation is not ethical, for instance when efficacy has been established in general terms, but where evidence in different clinical conditions has to be assessed. Another example is ascertainment of rare but serious adverse events, where even meta-analyses could lack sufficient numbers of patients or events.

SEARCHING

To examine the amount of evidence, PubMed was searched for original studies of two main types - randomised studies not included in the systematic review for some reason, and for any cohort or cross sectional studies - involving sildenafil, tadalafil, and vardenafil published between 2000 and 2005. Tables of the studies are not shown here for reasons of space, but are available on the Bandolier Internet site (www.ebandolier.com).

RANDOMISED STUDIES NOT INCLUDED IN SYSTEMATIC REVIEWS

Ten sildenafil studies with 561 patients were not included in a recent systematic review. All were randomised, and three were double blind. One was a withdrawal design demonstrating that beneficial effects of sildenafil were lost on stopping the drug, one in Parkinson's disease where hypotension stopped the study, and one crossover study in congestive heart failure.

The other studies were either declared to be open, or were not convincingly double blind. These studies from Europe and Central and South America were mostly small, with seven having fewer than 50 patients. Two of the larger and two of the smaller studies compared sildenafil directly with apomorphine or phentolamine, and found sildenafil to be more effective.

One study was found for tadalafil, with 4,262 patients in a European study examining dosing preferences. No such studies were found for vardenafil.

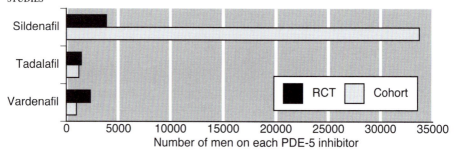

Number of men on each PDE-5 inhibitor

COHORT OR CROSS-SECTIONAL STUDIES

Twenty-five sildenafil studies with 33,708 patients were found. There were 17 prospective cohort studies with 3,668 men, six retrospective cohorts with 29,352 men, and two cross-sectional studies with 127 men.

The prospective cohort studies were often large, and nine of them had more than 100 men. Almost all of them had measures of improvement in erectile function, most often using the standard IIEF outcomes. Improvement rates were typically above 70%, consistent with findings from the randomised trials.

With one exception, the retrospective studies had information on over 500 men each, with one having over 22,000 men. This UK study was designed to look for adverse events following the introduction of sildenafil in the UK, and is described in detail later.

For tadalafil there were two prospective cohorts with 1201 men, and for vardenafil two more cohorts with 964 men. In each case one of these was an open-label extension of randomised trials.

COMMENT

For cohort studies alone, there were almost ten times as many patients on sildenafil (33,708) as in the included randomised trials (under 4,000 in a recent systematic review). For tadalafil and vardenafil there was information from fewer men in cohort studies than in randomised trials (Figure 6.8).

What this shows, interestingly, is that for a new treatment in an area where previously there were few effective treatments available, we might expect to see a considerable amount of observational information published, which can be useful and probably should not be overlooked.

# SECTION 7

# OTHER TREATMENTS FOR ERECTILE DYSFUNCTION

CLINICAL BOTTOM LINE

Intraurethral alprostadil works, though there is not a large evidence-base from randomised trials. It is associated with penile pain, and occasionally with prolonged erections. It will not be a first-line treatment choice.

---

Alprostadil is a prostaglandin that can be used to treat erectile dysfunction. There are different methods of using it, by injection into the penis (intracavernosal), by inserting a pellet into the urethra (transurethral), or by a cream or gel applied to the glans penis (topical). This section looks at intracavernosal injection.

SEARCHING

Searching was done using PubMed, Medline and the Cochrane Library, up to September 2005. Randomised trials in which alprostadil was compared with placebo were sought. Details of the trials were abstracted and quality scoring done with a 5 point scale. For crossover or partial crossover designs, details of the first phase were used (as a parallel group trial) where possible, and where this was not possible the full crossover data was used.

The outcome sought was patient/partner judgement of satisfactory erections suitable for intercourse, or actual intercourse, at home. Ideally this was on a patient basis, rather than on event basis, which was a secondary outcome. Relative risk and NNT were calculated using standard methods.

RESULTS

Four randomised trials were found, one with a placebo comparison [1], two comparing intracavernosal with transurethral alprostadil [2,3], and one a comparison with sildenafil [4]. The trials were small, and varied in their outcomes, which often included laboratory as well as clinical results.

No pooled analysis was possible. These trials tell us that while intracavernosal alprostadil works, and probably works better than transurethral alprostadil, it is associated with high levels of penile pain, and some prolonged erections.

# COMMENT

Intracavernosal injection of alprostadil will not be the first treatment choice for all men with erectile dysfunction. It may be useful for some men in which other treatments do not work.

### REFERENCES:

1   Linet et al. Efficacy and safety of intracavernosal alprostadil in men with erectile dysfunction. NEJM 1996 334: 873-877.
2   Shokeir et al. Intracavernosal versus intraurethral alprostadil: a prospective randomized study. BJU International 1999 83: 812-815.
3   Shabsigh et al. Intracavernosal alprostadil Alfadex is more efficacious, better tolerated, and preferred over intraurethral alprostadil plus optional Actis: a comparative, randomized, crossover, multicentre study. Urology 2000 55: 109-113.
4   Mancini et al. Sildenafil citrate vs intracavernosal alprostadil for patients with arteriogenic erectile dysfunction: a randomised placebo controlled study. International Journal of Impotence Research 2004 16: 8-12.

# Topical Alprostadil

## Clinical bottom line

Topical alprostadil works, though there is not a large evidence-base from randomised trials. It is associated with genital burning for man and partner.

---

Alprostadil is a prostaglandin that can be used to treat erectile dysfunction. This section looks at topical application.

## Searching

Searching was done using PubMed, Medline and the Cochrane Library, up to September 2005. Randomised trials in which alprostadil was compared with placebo were sought. Details of the trials were abstracted and quality scoring done with a 5 point scale. For crossover or partial crossover designs, details of the first phase were used (as a parallel group trial) where possible, and where this was not possible the full crossover data was used.

The outcome sought was patient/partner judgement of satisfactory erections suitable for intercourse, or actual intercourse, at home. Ideally this was on a patient basis, rather than on event basis, which was a secondary outcome. Relative risk and NNT were calculated using standard methods.

## Results

One laboratory study [1], and one meta-analysis of two randomised trials (published twice [2,3]) were found. Studies were not large, nor were they of long duration. Higher doses of topical alprostadil clearly work with penetration enhancers, though penile erythema for men and vaginal burning for partners may be a problem.

## Comment

There is only limited evidence concerning the efficacy of topical alprostadil.

### References

1    I Goldstein et al. A double-blind, placebo-controlled, efficacy and safety study of topical gel formulation of 1% alprostadil (Topiglan) for the in-office treatment of erectile dysfunction. Urology 2001 57: 301-305.

2   C Steidle et al. Topical alprostadil cream for the treatment of erectile dysfunction: a combined analysis of the phase II program. Urology 2002 60: 1077-1082.

3   H Padma-nathan et al. The efficacy and safety of a topical alprostadil cream, Alprodex-TD, for the treatment of erectile dysfunction: two phase 2 studies in mild-to-moderate and severe ED. International Journal of Impotence Research 2003 15: 10-17.

# Transurethral Alprostadil

## Clinical bottom line

Transurethral alprostadil has been tested in men with erectile dysfunction at home. All three trials have used enriched enrolment, and data pooling was not possible because outcomes were reported using men and attempts at intercourse as denominators. It would appear that over 50% of men who have previously responded to alprostadil can achieve successful intercourse at home with transurethral alprostadil. The NNT calculated on an intention to treat basis was 3.5 (3.1 to 4.0) for one man to achieve successful intercourse at home who would not have done so with placebo. Penile pain was relatively common, but usually described as mild.

---

Alprostadil is a prostaglandin that can be used to treat erectile dysfunction. There are different methods of using it, by injection into the penis (intracavernosal), by inserting a pellet into the urethra (transurethral), or by a cream or gel applied to the glans penis (topical). This review covers transurethral application, and studies comparing transurethral with intracavernosal injection are dealt with in the section on intracavernosal injection.

## Searching

Searching was done using PubMed, Medline, and the Cochrane Library, to September 2005. Randomised trials in which alprostadil was compared with placebo were sought. Details of the trials were abstracted and quality scoring done with a 5 point scale. For crossover or partial crossover designs, details of the first phase were used (as a parallel group trial) where possible, and where this was not possible the full crossover data was used.

The outcome sought was patient/partner judgement of satisfactory erections suitable for intercourse, or actual intercourse, at home. Ideally this was on a patient basis, rather than on event basis, which was a secondary outcome. Relative risk and NNT were calculated using standard methods.

## Results

Three trials [1-3] were found in which outcomes at home were measured; quality scores were 2 or 3 out of 5 points. All used enriched enrolment, in which the home trial only took place when a man had been shown to respond to alprostadil in clinic with an erection of sufficient rigidity for intercourse.

At least half the time a successful erection that allowed intercourse resulted from use of transurethral alprostadil at home in men in whom it had already been shown to work in the clinic. Penile pain was relatively common, but usually described as mild.

| Analysis | Successful intercourse with | | Relative benefit (95% CI) | NNT (95% CI) |
| | Alprostadil Number/Total (%) | Placebo Number/Total (%) | | |
| --- | --- | --- | --- | --- |
| Per protocol | 345/553 (62%) | 101/58(17) | 3.6 (3.0 to 4.4) | 2.2 (2.0 to 2.5) |
| Intention to treat | 345/856 (40) | 101/885 (10) | 3.5 (2.9 to 4.3) | 3.5 (3.1 to 4.0) |

We can calculate the NNT for a man to have one successful intercourse at least once at home with alprostadil compared with placebo. This can be done on the basis of a per protocol calculation, using the numbers randomised at enriched enrolment. Alternatively, if we accept that those enrolled but not randomised were treatment failures and would have been equally randomised between alprostadil and placebo groups, we can calculate an intention to treat NNT. The calculations are given in Table 7.1.

The relative benefit remains the same, but the NNT rises substantially with the intention to treat calculation, from two men to four men needing to be treated for one to have successful intercourse at home who would not have with placebo.

## COMMENT

What is remarkable is that the references found on searching (below) were many. The trials at home with useful outcomes were relatively few, and even these may not extrapolate to everyday practice. For instance, in the largest study (Padma-Nathan et al), about one third of the men originally enrolled did not respond in the clinic, or for some other reason did not participate in the at-home trial, with a similar proportion in the Williams trial. In these two studies 1155 men entered the at-home trials out of 1760 originally enrolled. This limits the application of these results, though perhaps the intention to treat calculation becomes more useful.

It is interesting also to visit alprostadil in the round, as it were, and compare this report with the original report in Bandolier, which was somewhat more enthusiastic in those early days. A Cochrane review [4] covers similar ground.

REFERENCES:

1    WJ Hellstrom et al. A double-blind, placebo-controlled evaluation of the erectile response to transurethral alprostadil. Urology 1996 48:851-856.
2    H Padma-Nathan et al. Treatment of men with erectile dysfunction with transurethral alprostadil. NEJM 1997 336: 1-7.

3   G Williams  et al. Efficacy and safety of transurethral alprostadil therapy in men with erectile dysfunction. MUSE Study Group. British Journal of Urology 1998 81: 889-894.

4   R Urciuoli et al. Prostaglandin E1 for treatment of erectile dysfunction. Cochrane Database of Systematic Reviews 2004 issue 2.

# SUBLINGUAL APOMORPHINE FOR ERECTILE DYSFUNCTION

## CLINICAL BOTTOM LINE

Sublingual apomorphine is effective in erectile dysfunction. The number needed to treat compared with placebo for erections sufficient for intercourse was 7 (5 to 10). Nausea was the chief adverse effect.

---

Apomorphine is a centrally acting, nonopioid, dopamine agonist. Such agents are known to cause erections in rats, and dopamine agonists improve erections in men treated for Parkinson's disease. The chief problem is nausea.

## SEARCHING

Searching was done using PubMed, Medline and the Cochrane Library, up to September 2005. Randomised trials in which apomorphine was compared with placebo or other treatments were sought. Details of the trials were abstracted and quality scoring done with a 5 point scale.

The outcome sought was patient/partner judgement of satisfactory erections suitable for intercourse, or actual intercourse, at home. Relative risk and NNT were calculated using standard methods.

## RESULTS

### PLACEBO COMPARISON

Four studies [1-4], scoring mainly 4 on the quality scale compared sublingual apomorphine at various fixed or dose-optimised systems between 2 and 6 mg with placebo, in 1594 men. A successful outcome, usually as percentage of successful attempts at intercourse, occurred in 45% of men with apomorphine, compare with 29% of men with placebo (Figure 7.1).

The relative risk was 1.4 (95% CI 1.2 to 1.7), and the number needed to treat was 6.6 (5.0 to 9.6).

FIGURE 7.1: SUBLINGUAL APOMORPHINE COMPARED WITH PLACEBO

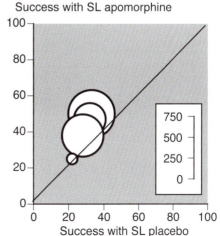

Success with SL apomorphine

Success with SL placebo

Two studies [5,6] scoring 2 on the quality scale compared sublingual apomorphine with oral sildenafil in open studies. In the larger of these, using titrated dosing to effect, sublingual apomorphine was much less effective than sildenafil.

### ADVERSE EVENTS

In all these studies, nausea was the commonest adverse event with apomorphine.

## COMMENT

While apomorphine is effective, in that it is better than placebo, it is clearly less effective than oral PDE-5 inhibitors.

### REFERENCES

1    E Dula et al. Efficacy and safety of fixed-dose and dose-optimization regimens of sublingual apomorphine versus placebo in men with erectile dysfunction. Urology 2000 56: 130-135.

2    E Dula et al. Double-blind, crossover comparison of 3 mg apomorphine SL with placebo and with 4 mg apomorphine SL in male erectile dysfunction. European Urology 2001 39: 558-563.

3    AT von Keitz et al. A European multicentre study to evaluate the tolerability of apomorphine sublingual administered in a forced dose-escalation regimen in patients with erectile dysfunction. BJU International 2002 89: 409-415.

4    P Gontero et al. Clinical efficacy of apomorphine SL in erectile dysfunction of diabetic men. International Journal of Impotence of Research 2005 17: 80-85.

5    I Eardley et al. An open-label, randomized, flexible-dose, crossover study to assess the comparative efficacy and safety of sildenafil citrate and apomorphine hydrochloride in men with erectile dysfunction. BJU International 2004 93: 1271-1275.

6    P Perimenis et al. Efficacy of apomorphine and sildenafil in men with nonarteriogenic erectile dysfunction. A comparative crossover study. Andrologica 2004 36: 106-110.

## CLINICAL BOTTOM LINE

There is limited information about the oral or intracavernosal use of phentolamine, alone or in combination with intracavernosal papaverine. An effect seems to be shown, but in such small numbers of patients (137 men) that it would be unwise to extrapolate from these results. For intracavernosal phentolamine plus papaverine the NNT was 2.1 (1.6 to 3.2) in 93 men in trials conducted in the 1980s. There was one case of priapism.

---

## SEARCHING

Searching was done using PubMed, Medline and the Cochrane Library, up to September 2005. Randomised trials in which phentolamine was compared with placebo were sought. Details of the trials were abstracted and quality scoring done with a 5 point scale. For crossover or partial crossover designs, details of the first phase were used (as a parallel group trial) where possible, or the full crossover data was used.

The outcome sought was patient/partner judgement of satisfactory erections suitable for intercourse, or actual intercourse, at home. Ideally this was on a patient basis, rather than on event basis, which was a secondary outcome. Relative risk and NNT were calculated using standard methods.

## RESULTS

### PLACEBO-CONTROLLED TRIALS

Searching unearthed three papers from 1987 [1-3], with quality scores of 2 or 3 out of 5. One [1] examined oral phentolamine at three doses compared to placebo in 40 men. On these small numbers the only sensible conclusion was that there was an apparent effect.

Two studies on intracavernosal phentolamine plus papaverine [2,3] showed larger effects in somewhat more men. Overall 23/47 men (49%, 95% CI 35-63%) achieved erections adequate for intercourse with the combination. In contrast, 1/47 men (2%, 95% CI 0-6%) achieved the same outcome with saline placebo. These were the same men in crossover trials. The relative benefit was 16 (3.2 to 77) and the NNT was 2.1 (1.6 to 3.2).

### ACTIVE CONTROLLED TRIALS

Two randomised active controlled trials were found. One [4] compared intracavernous sodium nitroprusside with papaverine phentolamine in 42 men, and measured penile

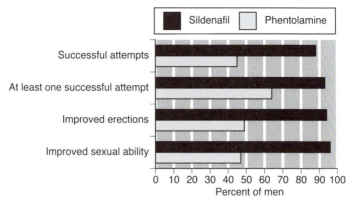

length, circumference and hardness, and found no major differences.

Another randomised open-label study [5] compared 123 men given sildenafil (25-100 mg) with 119 men given oral phentolamine 40 mg, to a maximum of one tablet daily, for eight weeks. Efficacy was assessed using IIEF questionaires at baseline and end of the study, together with global questions about efficacy.

The results for sildenafil were much better than those for phentolamine in these men, who had an average age of 55 years and average duration of erectile dysfunction of more than three years. The average number of successful attempts per week was much higher (3.1) for sildenafil than for phentolamine (1.7), and other outcomes also were much better (Figure 7.2).

COMMENT

There really isn't a great weight of evidence here, with 40 men on oral phentolamine and 48 using an intracavernosal combination in placebo-controlled trial. The one active controlled trial comparing oral phentolamine with oral sildenafil was open, but large, and showed phentolamine to be significantly less effective. These small numbers tell us nothing sensible about adverse events, though one case of priapism was found, and some cases of mild reaction at the injection site.

REFERENCES

1    AJ Becker et al. Oral phentolamine as treatment for erectile dysfunction. Journal of Urology 1998 159: 1214-1216.
2    TC Gasser et al. Intracavernous self-injection with phentolamine and papaverine for the treatment of impotence. Journal of Urology 1987 137: 678-680.
3    EA Kiely et al. Penile function following intracavernosal injection of vasoactive agents or saline. British Journal of Urology1987 59: 473-476.

4   F Ugarte et al. Comparison of the efficacy and safety of sildenafil citrate (Viagra) and oral phentyolamine for the treatment of erectile dysfunction. International Journal of Impotence Research 2002 14 Suppl 2: S48-S53.

5   Q Fu et al. A clinical comparative study on effects of intracavernous injection of sodium nitroprusside and papaverine/phentolamine in erectile dysfunction patients. Asian Journal of Urology 2000 2: 301-303.

# Testosterone for Erectile Dysfunction

## Clinical Bottom Line

There is limited evidence that testosterone can help men with erectile dysfunction. In five randomised comparisons with placebo in 109 men, testosterone was better than placebo in four, and the overall NNT was 2.1 (1.5 to 3.0). There is good evidence that testosterone supplementation works best in men with initial serum testosterone concentrations below 12 nmol/L, and is ineffective in men with serum testosterone concentrations above this.

Information on trial quality is limited, and this result has insufficient weight to drive clinical practice.

---

## Systematic Reviews

Two systematic reviews were found, from 2000 and 2005.

### Review 1 [Jain et al, 2000]

The first review sought papers in which testosterone was given as the only method of therapy for erectile dysfunction. Included studies had to have a clear and quantifiable measure of erectile response, rather than desire, and include a number of measures like surveys and patient diaries. Electronic databases were searched, with the date of the last search in 1998.

Formal evaluation of trial quality was not performed, and randomised and case control studies were included.

### Results

Overall, 16 studies were included, but we are told only that five trials (from 1979 to 1994) with 109 patients were randomised, and had comparison to placebo. The results of those trials are shown in Figure 7.3.

With placebo, 9/54 men had a response (eight in one trial). The percentage response was 17% (95% CI 7-27). For testosterone 36/55 men had a response (65%, 95% CI 53%-78%). The relative benefit was about 4 (because of zero or 100% val-

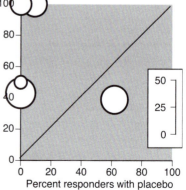

FIGURE 7.3: L'ABBÉ PLOT OF ERECTILE RESPONDERS TO TESTOSTERONE AND PLACEBO

Percent responders with testosterone

Percent responders with placebo

98

ues in many cells, accurate computation is impossible). The NNT for one man to have a response with testosterone compared with placebo was 2.1 (1.5 to 3.0). Adverse events were not described.

## REVIEW 2 [ISIDORI ET AL, 2005]

The second review sought randomised trials only, and only six of the 16 studies in the first review were included in the second review. Information was abstracted from trials for a range of outcomes, including serum testosterone levels at baseline and after treatment. The analysis used standardised mean differences, so that simple explanations of the results were not easy.

### RESULTS

Searching found 17 papers, 14 of which were both randomised and blind. Five studies were on hypogonadal men (testosterone below 7 nmol/L, seven on eugonadal men (testosterone above 12 nmol/L), and five on mixed types. There were 656 men, with 284 randomised to testosterone, 274 to placebo, and 88 in crossover design studies. Overall the mean age was 58 years. Most studies had fewer than 20 men in each trial arm. There were large differences in testosterone preparation used, dosing, delivery method, and prevalence of sexual dysfunction at baseline.

In studies with baseline testosterone below 10 nmol/L, with between three and six studies reporting outcomes, testosterone significantly improved:

- morning erections
- erectile function
- intercourse frequency
- sexual motivation
- sexual satisfaction
- sexual thoughts
- total erections

In studies with baseline testosterone above 10 nmol/L, results were much less impressive, with less difference between testosterone and placebo, and with significance only for:

- morning erections
- intercourse frequency
- sexual thoughts
- total erections

There was some, limited, evidence that no effect was found in men with baseline testosterone above 12 nmol/L, and that for both libido and erectile function the magnitude of effect was inversely related to the baseline testosterone concentration in the study population: men with lower testosterone did better.

## COMMENT

These would make useful teaching papers. The first review tries to do many things, and probably fails to meet many of the standards we look for in meta-analyses while remaining enthusiastic, and interesting, and even possibly relevant. The second review is much better in that it was of mainly randomised and blind studies, but they were small, and some of the extrapolations are limited in their utility.

There is also the issue of searching efficiency. Some studies in the second, later, review were not found by the first, earlier, review, even though they were published at that time. At least two small trials were available for the second review, but not included, when they perhaps might have been (though they were too small to have changed any results). We should not be censorious, because in recent years searching has improved, and labelling of trials has improved considerably.

The main problem is one of numbers. There just weren't enough to make any sense, despite attempts to analyse, for instance, the relative efficacy of different modes of testosterone delivery. For what it's worth, transdermal application seemed better than others, and not scrotal administration or intramuscular injection.

These reviews give a reasonable idea of where we are now, and what the literature is. Useful if we were considering testosterone development, or if all other acceptable treatments had failed.

### REFERENCES

1   P Jain et al. Testosterone supplementation for erectile dysfunction: results of a meta-analysis. Journal of Urology 2000 164: 371-375.
2   AM Isidori et al. Effects of testosterone on sexual function in men: results of a meta-analysis. Clinical Endocrinology 2005 63: 381-394.

# Trazodone for Erectile Dysfunction

## Clinical bottom line

There is no good evidence that trazodone is effective for erectile dysfunction.

---

A number of reviews about male sexual dysfunction mention the use of trazodone for maintaining erections. Many Internet sites about male sexual dysfunction also mention trazodone as a specific treatment, and some give it as much weight as treatments like sildenafil and the newer phosphodiesterase inhibitors. It is clearly important to have a variety of possible treatments, especially as erectile dysfunction may have several causes. A systematic review [1] informs us how little we actually know about trazodone for this indication.

## Systematic review

Searching included MEDLINE, the Cochrane Library and specialised registries of trials. For inclusion trials had to include men with erectile dysfunction and be randomised trials comparing trazodone with placebo or other control, have outcomes related to erectile dysfunction and last at least one week. The primary outcome was successful sexual intercourse attempts. Additional literature searches to September 2005 found no more RCTs.

## Results

Five trials with 240 men reported trazodone therapy compared with placebo. The dose of trazodone was 50 mg daily in one trial, and 150-200 mg daily in the other four. Duration was four weeks in four trials and 13 weeks in one. Two studies were from Turkey, and one each from Holland, Belgium and the USA. Most men in the trials had erectile dysfunction of at least three to six months' duration.

Four trials had outcomes, but only one of these had the primary outcome the authors sought, of successful sexual intercourse attempts. The other three had less well defined outcomes for improvement. The results are shown in Figure 7.4. Overall, with trazodone

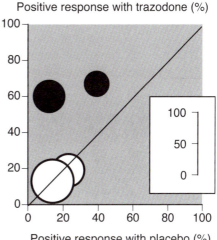

FIGURE 7.4: POSITIVE RESPONSE TO TREATMENT WITH TRAZODONE AND PLACEBO

Positive response with trazodone (%)

Positive response with placebo (%)

38/104 men (37%) improved, compared with 21/106 men (20%) with placebo. The results were better for the two trials (dark symbols in Figure 7.4) in which men had psychogenic erectile dysfunction, than in the two trials (light symbols) in which the erectile dysfunction had a physiological or mixed aetiology.

The authors of the paper decided *a priori* that the data were clinically heterogeneous, and used a random effects calculation for statistical significance. This concluded that overall there was no statistical improvement with trazodone (relative benefit 1.6; 95%CI 0.8 to 3.3). A less conservative approach using a fixed effects calculation would have shown statistical significance. For the two studies in men with psychogenic erectile dysfunction, the effect of trazodone again just about touched statistical significance, with 63% of men experiencing benefit with trazodone and 23% with placebo. The numbers were small (89 men in two trials), but the effect was large, with an imputed NNT of about 2.5.

### ADVERSE EVENTS

Adverse events were more frequent with trazodone than with placebo, but failed to reach statistical significance for any one adverse event. Sedation and dry mouth were common, and there was one case of priapism with trazodone. Adverse events or all-cause discontinuations were the same for both trazodone and placebo, at about 9%.

### COMMENT

We have here a nicely done review that leaves us without a definite conclusion because the information it found was just not good enough. The trials were small. They recruited men with different aetiologies for their erectile dysfunction. The outcomes were poorly defined, especially given what we have come to expect from modern research into erectile dysfunction. Trials were also generally of short duration. The best we can say is that we don't know enough. The next best is that we have a hint, and no more than a hint, that trazodone may be useful in men with erectile dysfunction of psychogenic aetiology.

What we have is a nice example of what happens in the early stages of a therapy being used for a different indication. Trials are small and the questions posed and answers obtained are diffuse. There is some evidence, and there may even be a biology, as priapism is a known rare adverse effect of trazodone. What we do not have is enough evidence to make unequivocal decisions. How this limited evidence can be used is simple. With much caution and after a great deal of thought, and for specific reasons in specific patients, or perhaps not at all until better evidence is available.

### REFERENCE:

1.  HA Fink et al. Trazodone for erectile dysfunction: a systematic review and meta-analysis. BJU International 2003 92: 441-446.

# Vacuum Constriction Devices for Erectile Dysfunction

## Clinical Bottom Line

There is little good randomised trial data on the use of vacuum constriction devices.

---

## Background

Vacuum constriction devices (VCDs) have been used for some time to increase blood flow to the penis and to achieve an erection. There is limited randomised trial evidence concerning VCDs, though there is a literature from the early-mid 1990s discussing their use, and the Raina paper contains useful references. VCDs have changed since then, and the present review looks at material from the late 1990s.

## Searching

Searching was done using PubMed, Medline and the Cochrane Library, up to September 2005. Randomised trials in which VCDs were compared with any other treatments were sought. Details of the trials were abstracted and quality scoring done with a 5 point scale.

The outcome sought was patient/partner judgement of satisfactory erections suitable for intercourse, or actual intercourse, at home. Relative risk and NNT were calculated using standard methods.

## Results

Only two randomised trials were found, both small, and both open studies.

In the Wylie study [1] 370 patients attending a specialist psychosexual service with psychogenic or combined aetiology for their ED had treatment choices including medication, intracavernosal injections, vacuum devices or psychotherapy. The couple psychotherapy option was chosen by 45 (12%).

Therapy was a package of relationship therapy and modified Masters and Johnson sex therapy, lasting 45 minutes occurring every two weeks, and modified for each couple. Half the men were randomly offered the concurrent use of a VCD (Rapport SM2000). The primary outcome was the sex therapist's assessment of response to treatment.

Of 25 randomised to VCD, 20 actually used it. Of these, 21 had moderate or good improvement (84%). Of 20 randomised to control, 12 (60%) had the same response. Few men chose to continue with the VCD, and most subsequently chose, and benefited from, medical therapy.

The Raina study [2] reports on 109 men randomised to VCD or no therapy for nine months after radical prostatectomy. Of 74 men randomised to VCD (53 with nerve sparing surgery), 60 actually used it, with constriction bands for intercourse, with a frequency of vaginal intercourse of twice per week. Of these 60, 10 reported a return of natural erections at a mean interval of nine months.

Thirty-one men were unsatisfied, and were instructed to take sildenafil 100 mg 1-2 hours before use of the device, and these men had additional benefits.

## COMMENT

There are few randomised trials of VCDs, though a number of case series have been reported. It is clearly successful for some men, but how it compares with medical therapy for particular causes of erectile dysfunction is uncertain. Vacuum constriction devices may be used commonly, and may work, but the evidence from randomised trials is limited.

REFERENCES:

1    KR Wylie et al. The potential benefit of vacuum devices augmenting psychosexual therapy for erectile dysfunction: a randomised controlled trial. Journal of Sex and Marital Therapy 2003 29: 227-236.
2    R Raina et al. Sildenafil citrate and vacuum constriction device combination enhances sexual satisfaction in erectile dysfunction after radical prostatectomy. Urology 2005 65: 360-364.

# VIP for Erectile Dysfunction

## Clinical Bottom Line

There is no evidence that intracavernosal vasoactive intestinal peptide (VIP) is effective. Intracavernosal VIP combined with phentolamine appears to have promise based on the results from one trial.

---

## Searching

Searching was done using PubMed, Medline and the Cochrane Library, up to September 2005. Randomised trials in which VIP was compared with placebo were sought. Details of the trials were abstracted and quality scoring done with a 5 point scale. For crossover or partial crossover designs, details of the first phase were used (as a parallel group trial) where possible, and where this was not possible the full crossover data was used.

The outcome sought was patient/partner judgement of satisfactory erections suitable for intercourse, or actual intercourse, at home. Ideally this was on a patient basis, rather than on event basis, which was a secondary outcome. Relative risk and NNT were calculated using standard methods.

## Results

### Intracavernosal VIP

In one study [1] of 24 men with non vasculogenic erectile dysfunction, none of them achieved penile rigidity sufficient for intercourse with a series of intracavernosal injections of 200 or 400 pmol of VIP.

### Intracavernosal VIP plus phentolamine

Use of 25 µg VIP plus 1 mg or 2 mg phentolamine in a single intracavernosal injection achieved satisfactory erections suitable for intercourse in 74% of uses, compared with 13% with placebo in 1200 attempts in 105 men who entered a randomised trial (apparently published twice [2,3]) and used the treatment. The relative benefit was 5.9 (4.1 to 8.4) and the NNT was 1.6 (1.5 to 1.8).

Flushing was noted with 50% of injections. Other local adverse events were common, including bruising. There was a single case of priapism.

A treatment for which there is relatively little information, most particularly concerning adverse events. There is too little information on which to judge efficacy, and while an NNT has been calculated, it is not a robust estimate with this trial design, and is based on successful attempts, not on men achieving success with the treatment. It should not be used as a basis for making therapy choices.

REFERENCES:

1    JB Roy et al. A clinical trial of intracavernous vasoactive intestinal peptide to induce penile erection. Journal of Urology 1990 143:302-304.
2    WWDinsmore et al. Treating men with predominantly nonpsychogenic erectile dysfunction with intracavernosal vasoactive intestinal polypeptide and phentolamine mesylate in a novel auto-injector system: a multicentre double-blind placebo-controlled study. BJU International 1999 83 :274-279.
3    D Sandhu et al. A double blind, placebo controlled study of intracavernosal vasoactive intestinal polypeptide and phentolamine mesylate in a novel auto-injector for the treatment of non-psychogenic erectile dysfunction. International Journal of Impotence Research 1999 11: 91-97.

# YOHIMBINE FOR ERECTILE DYSFUNCTION

## CLINICAL BOTTOM LINE

Yohimbine has been tested against placebo in 10 randomised trials with 659 men. Yohimbine provided satisfactory erections in 30% of men compared with 14% with placebo. The NNT compared with placebo for one man to achieve satisfactory erections was 6.4 (4.6 to 11). Adverse events were generally mild, though some men withdrew from treatment because of them.

---

## SYSTEMATIC REVIEW

The review by Ernst and colleagues [1] was updated because there were more trials that could be added, and in order to calculate NNTs.

Additional searching was done using PubMed, Medline, and the Cochrane Library, up to September 2005. Randomised trials in which oral yohimbine was compared with placebo were sought. Details of the trials were abstracted and quality scoring done with a 5 point scale. For crossover or partial crossover designs, details of the first phase were used (as a parallel group trial) where possible, and where this was not possible the full crossover data was used.

• Date review completed: 2005

• Number of trials included: 10

• Number of patients: 658

• Control group: placebo

• Main outcomes: self-report of success (various methods)

Inclusion criteria were double-blind, randomised, placebo-controlled trials of yohimbine for erectile dysfunction; adequate statistical evaluation; score of at least 3 on the 5 point Oxford quality scale; any language; published and unpublished trials.

The outcome sought was patient/partner judgement of satisfactory erections suitable for intercourse, or actual intercourse, at home. Ideally this was on a patient basis, rather than on event basis, which was a secondary outcome. Relative risk and NNT were calculated using standard methods.

## RESULTS

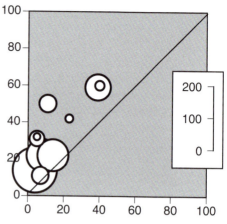

Ten trials were found, three more than in the Ernst review. There were 335 men receiving yohimbine and 324 receiving placebo. References to papers included and other references are in the reference table at the end of the article. The dose of yohimbine was between 15 mg and 40 mg daily, for 4-10 weeks of treatment. Details of the trials included in the analysis can be found on the Bandolier Internet site, together with references. Figure 7.5 shows a L'Abbé plot of the 10 trials.

Only one trial [2] showed a statistical benefit for yohimbine plus trazodone over placebo in 63 men. Overall, 99/335 men achieved satisfactory erections with yohimbine (30%, with 95% CI 25% to 34%). By contrast 45/324 men achieved satisfactory erections with placebo (14%, with 95% confidence interval of 10% to 18%).

Six men would have to be treated with yohimbine for one man to achieve satisfactory erections who would not have achieved them with placebo. The NNT was 6.4 (95%CI 4.6 to 11), and The relative benefit was 2.1 (95% CI 1.6 to 2.9). Studies with daily doses of 20 mg or more gave the same NNT as those with doses of 18 mg or less.

## COMMENT

The trials in this review were generally small, with only one studying as many as 100 men. With only 658 men in the trials, and 335 receiving yohimbine, this body of evidence is incomplete both as regards efficacy, and more especially as regards adverse events. Some studies mentioned serious adverse events, like hypertensive crisis or palpitations. There were a number of withdrawals on yohimbine, though a number of studies made no mention of adverse events.

### REFERENCE:

1   E Ernst, MH Pittler. Yohimbine for erectile dysfunction: a systematic review and meta-analysis of randomized clinical trials. Journal of Urology 1998; 159:433-436.
2   F Montorsi et al. Effect of yohimbine-trazodone on psychogenic impotence: a randomized, double-blind, placebo-controlled study. Urology 1994 44(5):732-736.